Fetal Monitoring in Practice

Second Edition

Donald Gibb
MD, MRCP, FRCOG

formerly Director of Women's Services
Consultant Obstetrician and Gynaecologist
Honorary Senior Lecturer
King's College School of Medicine and Dentistry
King's College Hospital
London

Sabaratnam Arulkumaran
PhD, FRCS(Ed), FRCOG

Professor
Department of Obstetrics and Gynaecology
University of Nottingham and
formerly Professor and Head
Department of Obstetrics and Gynaecology
National University Hospital
National University of Singapore
Kent Ridge
Singapore

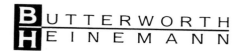
BUTTERWORTH
HEINEMANN

Butterworth-Heinemann
Linacre House, Jordan Hill, Oxford OX2 8DP
225 Wildwood Avenue, Woburn, MA 01801-2041
A division of Reed Educational and Professional Publishing Ltd

℞ A member of the Reed Elsevier plc group

OXFORD   AUCKLAND   BOSTON
JOHANNESBURG   MELBOURNE   NEW DELHI

First published 1992
Reprinted 1992 (twice), 1993 (three times), 1994 (twice), 1996, 1997
Second edition 1997
Reprinted 1998 (twice), 1999 (three times), 2000, 2001

British Library Cataloguing in Publication Data
A catalogue record for this book is available from the British Library

Library of Congress Cataloguing in Publication Data
A catalogue record for this book is available from the Library of Congress

ISBN 0 7506 3432 4

For information on all Butterworth-Heinemann publications
visit our website at www.bh.com

Composition by Genesis Typesetting, Rochester, Kent
Printed and bound in Great Britain by MPG Books Ltd, Bodmin, Cornwall

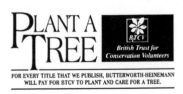

FOR EVERY TITLE THAT WE PUBLISH, BUTTERWORTH-HEINEMANN
WILL PAY FOR BTCV TO PLANT AND CARE FOR A TREE.

Contents

Foreword

The enduring challenge of obstetrics lies in the need to care for two people simultaneously. One, the mother, can express her feelings, answer our questions and allow us to examine her. The other, the fetus, is hidden far from our view and such information as we can obtain must be gained by resort to indirect methods. Until two or three decades ago such methods were primitive and crude but during that time they have seen rapid development and ever increasing sophistication. The birth process has been described as the most dangerous journey most of us are ever likely to make and it is expected nowadays that hazards and problems during that journey should be promptly recognized so as to allow suitable corrective action.

The objectives of fetal monitoring are simply stated. They are to ensure that any harm which might threaten the fetus in utero can be recognized in time to allow removal of the harmful influence or removal of the fetus from its hostile environment. This applies both during pregnancy and during labour. Drs Gibb and Arulkumaran are not only highly regarded academics in the field of perinatal medicine, they are both dynamic clinicians who have studied pregnancy and labour at first hand and in real depth. They bring a genuine authority to the subject of fetal monitoring in practice and have written with maturity and commendable common sense on this very important and complex subject. The deeper understanding which this volume will give to its readers will bring real benefits to their clinical practice. They have dedicated this work to the health of the mothers and babies who will surely be the beneficiaries of their efforts.

Professor AA Calder MD, FRCS(Edin), FRCP(Glas & Edin), FRCOG
Department of Obstetrics and Gynaecology
The Centre for Reproductive Biology
University of Edinburgh, UK

Preface

In promoting safe motherhood as espoused by the World Health Organization, our objectives must be to optimize the:

- health of the mother
- health of the offspring
- emotional satisfaction of the mother and her family.

In developing countries, with high maternal and perinatal mortality rates, limited resources and circumstances dictate that efforts are directed primarily at the first two objectives. In more developed countries with less frequent mortality attention can also be focused on the third goal.

The birth of a healthy baby is a universal aim. Although being born too early is the most common cause of perinatal loss, lack of oxygenation and nutrition is also a critical factor. Commonly referred to antenatally as intrauterine growth retardation and intrapartum as fetal distress this condition presents a great challenge to obstetricians. However, in spite of technological developments in ultrasound and electronic fetal monitors, there has been some disillusion with the results of clinical application. Unexpectedly small babies are born with asphyxia, normal-size babies are born asphyxiated and normal-size babies are delivered operatively for 'fetal distress' in excellent condition. Those who believe in electronic fetal heart rate monitoring are often reminded by the sceptics that randomized controlled trials have failed to show any benefits of the procedure. There have been several controlled trials some considering low-risk cases only and others taking high-risk and low-risk. Other trials have complemented electronic monitoring with pH measurement. Consistency of interpretation of the tracings agreed prospectively has not been a major feature of these studies. There is no consensus on how the procedure should be performed, the interpretation of results and the appropriate steps to be taken when the test is abnormal. Under such conditions the validity of such trials must be open to question. Of those studies only the Dublin Study[1] and that by Leveno et al. (1986)[2] consisted of large enough numbers to reach meaningful conclusions. The Dublin Study was performed on a selected population where only one-third of the intrapartum and neonatal deaths were included: preterm babies less than 29 weeks' gestation, cases with meconium-stained amniotic fluid, absent amniotic fluid and those who progressed rapidly in labour were excluded. Furthermore only 80% allocated to the electronically monitored group were monitored and 11% had uninterpretable traces. Leveno et al.[2] compared selective versus routine monitoring and showed no significant difference except a slightly higher caesarean section rate in routinely monitored cases. These studies highlight the need to identify the population to whom this technology should be applied. Intrapartum electronic fetal heart rate monitoring would not be expected to reduce a perinatal mortality rate because any effect would be swamped by deaths from other causes. Substantially less than one baby per 1000 births would be expected to die during labour under any circumstances. More subtle end-points need to be measured.

Technology in itself achieves nothing. It must be applied appropriately and correctly. Failure to understand this has resulted in the death of babies in spite of the intensive use of technology. Inappropriate application of technology and failure to take into account the clinical situation is common. The introduction of electronic fetal monitors has not been accompanied by any systematic attempt at education of the staff using them. The latter must be addressed and this is the prime objective of this book.

There is no such thing as 'no risk' in obstetrics. There is low-risk and high-risk, with a common phenomenon being a change in risk with time from the former to the latter; the converse does not occur. Excessive technology should not be applied to those who are manifestly at low-risk. It may confer no benefit, can generate both non-medical and medical anxiety and through subtle effects may cause significant harm. Women and their partners in developed societies sometimes seek natural childbirth (this really means birth with low technology and minimal intervention) and it is up to health service professionals to try to satisfy these needs. The unthinking application of technology is counter-productive. A relationship of trust and professionalism should bear fruit. It is acknowledged that the introduction of electronic fetal heart rate monitoring has contributed to an increase in the number of caesarean births. This is largely due to failure to understand the principles of the technique, but may also be attributed to a fear of litigation. Both can be effectively countered.

We believe an extensive effort in education is required. There are those who want to change the rules of the game before the previous rules have been agreed. We must beware of the enthusiasts for alternative methods such as Doppler ultrasonography, electrocardiographic waveform analysis, electromechanical intervals or whatever is their own personal interest at that time. It may be in their interest to decry fetal heart rate monitoring in order to supplant it. There is no evidence that any of these techniques are of superior or even equal value. Education to exploit fully the potential of fetal heart rate monitoring is the alternative, and through extensive involvement in the labour wards we are in a position to contribute to this. In the early 1980s we were privileged to be responsible for the deliveries under the care of the academic unit, Kandang Kerbau Hospital, Singapore. The total number of deliveries for the unit was 10 000 per year, with the government units supervising another 16 000 deliveries per year in the same labour ward. Epidural anaesthesia was not available; there was only one electronic fetal heart rate monitor and a considerable number of high-risk pregnancies. There were 28 beds in the high-risk delivery area and 18 beds in the low-risk delivery area. Ward rounds were no sooner finished than the next one started. More fetal monitors subsequently became available; however, there were never enough to monitor all of the mothers. Selection had to be undertaken and from this exercise we learned an enormous amount, through setting up clinical studies of selective electronic monitoring. The discipline of high profile involvement in the labour wards has continued in the hospitals where we now work. Daily consultant ward rounds, caesarean section reviews, perinatal death reviews and joint discussions with the neonatologists all contribute to greater understanding. Confidence is required, in knowing as much when not to intervene as when to intervene. In a climate of possible complaint and litigation, inexperienced junior staff must be taught how to make these decisions. Confidence to encourage the low-risk mother in pursuit of natural childbirth to have appropriate minimal technology will come with this knowledge. Good communication between staff and with the mother is an excellent method of avoiding complaint and litigation.

Women in the labour ward are looked after by a team of midwives and doctors. There should be no demarcation of midwives' cases and doctors' cases. Low-risk mothers in normal labour will be looked after largely by midwives and this should be encouraged with the inclusion of phlebotomy, intravenous cannula siting and perineal suturing. Continuity of care will be enhanced and job satisfaction promoted. High-risk women will have a greater degree of medical input extending to the anaesthetist, neonatologist and senior obstetricians. Paradoxically, low-risk women pursuing natural birth should meet the medical staff sooner rather than later and be assured of the back-up position. The doctor may be seen as a fire prevention officer rather than a firefighter summoned in a moment of crisis. A team approach with respect for the contribution of each

member will result in a healthy and productive working environment. Daily ward rounds and discussions form an important part of
this approach. This does not involve taking a group of strangers to
the bedside of a woman in labour; it involves meeting with the
midwives, discussing each woman's situation and seeing those who
need to be seen with the appropriate small group of immediate
providers of care.

The Government report, *Changing Childbirth* (1993), is an important challenge to the providers of care. It is not about power games
between doctors and midwives but about a true team approach to
woman-centred care. Midwives should have the responsibility of
continuity of care for the low-risk mother. All, however, bear the
responsibility for the safe passage of the baby. The midwives are in
the front line as they deliver most of the bedside care in the labour
ward. When the doctors become involved it is important that the
understanding and approach to fetal monitoring is consistent. It is
artificial to divorce the education of the medical staff from that of the
midwives. Midwives involved in caring for women in labour at
home have a special responsibility. They require special skills in the
application of clinical and low-technology monitoring.

The reforms of the National Health Service in the UK have critical
implications. Trust Hospital budgets and quality initiatives demand
attention is paid to Risk Management Programmes. Untoward
Clinical Incident reporting is in its infancy but is likely to assume
great importance. Early detailed statements from the staff involved
simplifies matters investigated at a later date and the importance of
legible, clear record-keeping does not require restating. Orientation
of new staff in these matters should be undertaken. Thus all new
staff in a labour ward should be provided with copies of the
guidelines and education in fetal monitoring. Copies of *Changing
Childbirth*, the *Confidential Enquiry into Maternal Mortality*, booklets
from the Stillbirth and Neonatal Death Society, and other relevant
documents should be freely available.

Case discussions and teaching sessions are very important.
Circumspection and tact are important elements in review of cases
with an adverse outcome. The aim is not to apportion blame but to
learn from the experience and hopefully prevent a similar outcome
in the future. Some of the examples in this book have been presented
to us at seminars we have conducted. These seminars, the
Kensington Seminars, have become very popular. The participants,
initially midwives but now including more doctors and legal
professionals, have said that we have discussed things they already
knew from experience but which they were not aware they knew.
This has been very satisfying and is the true meaning of 'education'.
We ourselves have learned a lot in a two-way process during such
discussions.

We hope that those reading this book will be stimulated and will learn something to help them in promoting safer childbirth. They will above all realize that their task is easier and, therefore, more satisfying than they have been previously led to believe. It was the philosopher, Goethe, who said: 'It annoys man that the truth is so simple'.

Acknowledgements

This book would not have been possible without extensive collaboration. Doctors and midwives in King's College Hospital, London, and the National University Hospital, Singapore, were always interested in collecting and discussing traces. Staff attending seminars all over the world but particularly at Kensington Town Hall, London brought traces and provoked discussion. Katie Morgan Adams and Gardenia Matley have run the organization Fetal Monitoring Education.

Oxford Sonicaid, Hewlett-Packard and Corometrics (Marquette Ltd) supplied equipment on generous terms. The Wellcome Institute Library, London gave permission for the reproduction of Figures 1.2 and 1.3.

Dr Jamal Zaidi collected traces. Mr Anthony Khoo in Singapore produced photographs. In London Alex Dionysiou prepared artwork, with Yvonne Bartlett and Barry Pike producing photographs.

Jayne White and Sue Gigney in London exercised enormous patience with the script. Dr Eko G Zhang checked and rechecked the manuscript of the second edition. Susan Devlin at Butterworth-Heinemann provided encouragement and on-going support.

Our families, Marie-Reine, Laurent and Pascale; Gayathri, Shankari, Nishkantha and Kailash, have tolerated our time-consuming obsession.

Thanks are expressed to all.

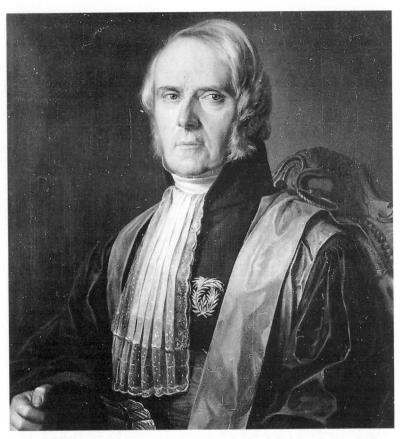

Figure 1.1 Jacques Alexandre de Kergaradec, robed as a Membre de l'Academie de Medicine Paris. (With thanks to Professor J. H. M. Pinkerton, Emeritus Professor of Midwifery and Gynaecology, Queen's University of Belfast)

Chapter 1

Introduction

No written records of the detection of fetal life in-utero exist in western literature until the 17th century. Around 1650 Marsac, a French physician, was ridiculed in a poem by a colleague Phillipe le Goust for claiming to hear the heart of the fetus 'beating like the clapper of a mill'. It was not until 1818 that Francois-Isaac, Mayor of Geneva, a forensic physician, reported the fetal heart audibly different from the maternal pulse heard by applying the ear directly to the pregnant mother's abdomen. Laennec, a physician working in Paris around 1816, was the father of the technique of auscultation of the adult heart and lungs. Le Jumeau, Vicomte de Kergaradec (Figure 1.1), also a physician working with Laennec, became interested in applying this technique to other conditions including pregnancy. John Creery Ferguson, later to become first Professor of Medicine at the Queen's University of Belfast, visited Paris meeting Laennec and Le Jumeau. On his return to Dublin in 1827, Ferguson was the first person in the British Isles to describe the fetal heart sounds. He influenced Evory Kennedy, assistant master at the Rotunda Lying-in Hospital in Dublin, who wrote his famous work entitled *Observations on Obstetric Auscultation* in 1833. There was much argument over the technique of listening, some demanding the use of the stethoscope for reasons of decency only. At that time some doctors examined pregnant women through their clothing and this respect for the modesty of the woman must have inhibited the spread of obstetric auscultation. Anton Friedrich Hohl was the first to describe the design of the fetal stethoscope in 1834 (Figure 1.2). Depaul modified this (Figure 1.3) describing both in his *Traite D'Auscultation Obstetricale* in 1847. Although Pinard's name is most commonly associated with the stethoscope his version followed several others, only appearing in 1876. Many papers were subsequently published in a variety of languages elaborating the technique. In 1849 Kilian proposed the 'stethoscopical indications for forceps operation': 'The forceps must be applied under favourable conditions without delay when the fetal heart tones diminish to less than 100 beats per minute (bpm) or when they increase to 180 bpm or when they lose their purity of tone'. Winkel, in 1893,

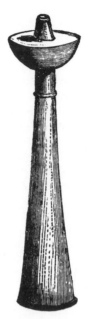

Figure 1.2   The Hohl fetal stethoscope (Wellcome Institute Library, London)

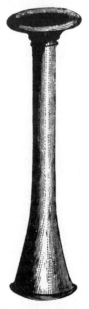

Figure 1.3   The Depaul fetal stethoscope (Wellcome Institute Library, London)

empirically set the limits of the normal heart rate at 120 bpm to 160 bpm. This has been carried forward for many years and reviewed in the light of the large amount of material produced by electronic recording.

If hearing the fetal heart was of any value then it was recognized that this was based on a very small sample of time subject to considerable observer variability. Listening for 15 seconds in 1 hour is only to sample 0.4% of the time. More continuous monitoring may be desirable. The advent of audiovisual technology associated with the development of the film industry in the early 20th century set the scene for technological developments that led to the equipment we have today. In 1953, while working in Lewisham Hospital, south-east London, Gunn and Wood reported 'The Amplification and Recording of Foetal Heart Sounds' in the *Proceedings of the Royal Society of Medicine*. In 1958, Hon pioneered electronic fetal monitoring in the USA. Caldeyro-Barcia in Uruguay and Hammacher in Germany reported their observations on the various heart rate patterns associated with fetal distress. This set the scene for the production of the first commercially available fetal monitor by Hammacher and Hewlett Packard in 1968 soon to be followed by Sonicaid in the UK. It is notable that Saling in Berlin had reported the use of fetal scalp blood sampling to study fetal pH 2 years prior to this in 1966. Fetal scalp blood pH assessment was developed in parallel with electronic monitoring, not as a sequel to it as might be assumed from our current practice.

The early equipment used phonocardiography, simply to listen and record sounds coming from the maternal abdomen as well as generating the fetal heart rate from the fetal electrocardiograph (ECG) from a fetal scalp electrode. Phonocardiography produces inferior traces because of the other extraneous sounds that confuse the picture. This problem was solved very quickly by the introduction of Doppler ultrasound transducers. When the Doppler transducer is applied to the maternal abdomen a Doppler signal is emitted in the direction of the fetal heart, the location of which has already been determined by auscultation. The signal is altered by a moving structure according to the Doppler shift principle and received by the transducer in its altered form. The moving structure is usually the moving heart and the blood flowing through it. Ultrasound Doppler technology has improved considerably in recent years and the latest generation of monitors produce excellent quality external traces, comparable to those generated by direct ECG. The previous justification that rupture of the membranes and application of a fetal electrode is necessary in order to generate a good quality trace is no longer valid. This improvement can be largely attributed to the technique of autocorrelation or dual autocorrelation and the use of wide beams. Monitoring of both twins externally has presented problems because of interference between the two Doppler beams. That has been solved in the latest equipment by the use of two different frequencies or the same frequency but distinguished by position using ultrasound 'windows' in the two ultrasound transducers so that the beams do not interfere with each other. The direct fetal ECG can be obtained by an external or internal technique. The external technique is only used in a research situation because the signal has to be electronically cleaned to remove the maternal ECG and electrical activity from the anterior abdominal wall. Direct detection of the fetal heart rate from a fetal electrode applied to the fetus at vaginal examination is used in clinical practice. This is commonly called a scalp electrode but is better termed a fetal electrode in view of its frequent application to the breech. All machines provide an external tocography facility through a relatively simple strain gauge transducer. It should be appreciated that this provides only an indirect assessment of the

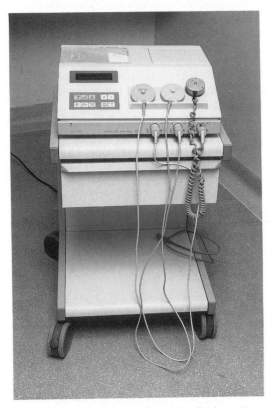

Figure 1.4   Oxford-Sonicaid Meridian fetal monitor

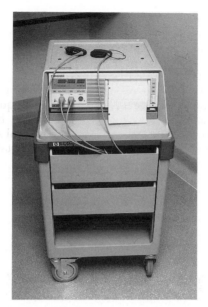

Figure 1.5   Hewlett Packard 1350 fetal monitor

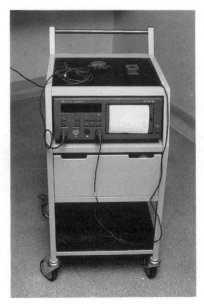

Figure 1.6   Corometrics 116 fetal monitor

uterine contractions. In the unusual situation of requiring direct data about the intrauterine pressure, an intrauterine catheter is necessary with the relevant option in the machine. However, the climate of childbirth has retreated from the excessive use of invasive technology and the role of internal monitoring has become much more limited.

The clinical needs should be assessed and the specification of the machine required determined accordingly. A monitor to be used for antenatal monitoring does not require the intrapartum options and is therefore less expensive. Most modern monitors (Figures 1.4–1.6) have similar specifications. The specification of a top of the range intrapartum monitor is shown in Table 1.1.

Table 1.1   Specification of an intrapartum monitor

Reliable
User friendly with operating manual and video
Robust with customized trolley

Fetal heart rate by external Doppler ultrasound (US) with autocorrelation
Fetal heart rate by fetal electrode (ECG)
Twin monitoring US and ECG
Twin monitoring US and US

Maternal heart rate
Event marker

External tocography
Internal tocography as an option

Mode, date and time printout
Keypad as an option

Automatic blood pressure, pulse and Po_2 facility (an option selectively for high-risk labours)

Antepartum monitors have become smaller. The Sonicaid Team (Figure 1.7) can be used with or without the printer module. Huntleigh (HNE Healthcare) has produced the Baby Dopplex (Figure 1.8) at low cost. Both Oxford Sonicaid and Huntleigh have produced new models of hand-held Doptones (Figure 1.9) which include a digital display of the heart rate. Some models are waterproof for use in the water-labour scenario. Low cost printers

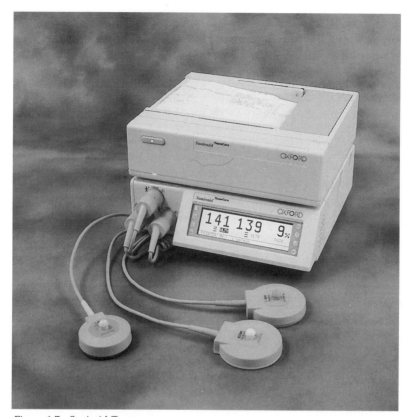

Figure 1.7   Sonicaid Team

which can be attached to such devices are being developed. Such systems offer exciting possibilities to countries that have not yet started on the troublesome journey of extensive electronic fetal monitoring. They must be helped to avoid the costly mistakes made by the more developed countries. Technology should be appropriate, low cost and high quality.

The value of telemetry and telephone transmission of the fetal heart rate (FHR) remains to be proven: investment should not be made in these options without a clear purpose. Telemetric transmission of the cardiotochograph (CTG) has become more practicable with improved technology in recent years, allowing the woman to remain mobile in early labour. However, more selective use of the technology has meant that some of the women who had telemetric monitoring do not actually require continuous electronic monitoring

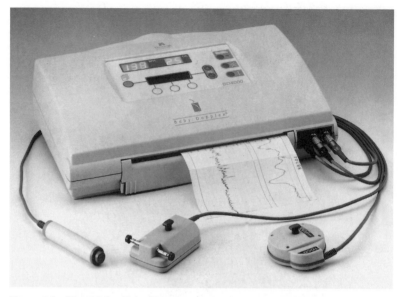

Figure 1.8   Huntleigh – Baby Dopplex

after the initial admission CTG (see later). The advent of mobile epidural anaesthesia and the use of water pools may rekindle the need for this kind of technology.

A solid trolley is an important investment to protect the machine during its busy life in the clinical area. Servicing, backup and supplies of paper and electrodes must be assured. At the time of writing the overall cost of a good quality monitor in the UK is about £9000 for an intrapartum monitor and £5000 for an antepartum monitor. Modern machines have been factory tested to ensure proper functioning in any climate in the world. They are designed to be used 24 hours a day, 7 days a week. Although the concept of rest and recovery is valid for human beings, it is not necessary for such machines!

An important step is to identify the midwifery and technical staff who will be responsible for day-to-day supervision and maintenance of this equipment. It is uncommon for such equipment to develop technical faults and defects will more often be user related. Simple housekeeping and in-service education will pay dividends. Not putting jelly on the tocograph transducer, not breaking the plugs by using push-pull rather than screw action, being careful that transducer cables are not run over and broken by trolley wheels (see Figure 1.4) and ensuring the use of the correct paper the right way

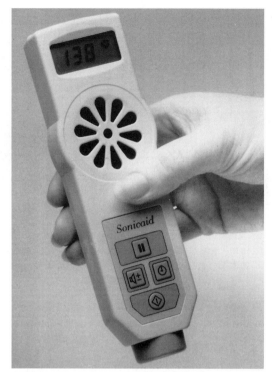

Figure 1.9   Hand-held Doppler

round are fairly simple instructions sometimes not given due attention. An expensive piece of equipment requires commonsense care. It is a pity if equipment is out of action because of user errors.

Chapter 2

Clinical assessment and recording

The process of birth is the most dangerous journey an individual undertakes. The complete journey is from conception until discharge from hospital of the healthy mother and baby. The continuum of fetal health involves antenatal well-being and neonatal well-being. This is the modern concept of perinatology. As few, if any, obstetricians are also neonatologists a clearer concept is maternofetal medicine. Although we are not neonatologists, we must maintain an interest in our *in utero* patient during his or her stay in the neonatal unit, just as the neonatologist will have joined us in assessment and counselling of the high-risk mother antenatally.

The part of the journey with which we are particularly concerned is that of labour and delivery. The concept of preparation is an important one and for our purposes we consider this journey to start with admission to the labour ward. When we prepare for a journey we ensure that we are in good health, our vehicle is in good condition, the roads we will drive on are safe and that we have a good insurance policy. Admission to the labour ward is the time for such a review of the pregnant mother. Intrapartum events are a continuum of antenatal events. Many babies who get into difficulty in labour have already become compromised in the antenatal period and our surveillance system must be designed to find these fetuses and ensure their safe delivery. Assessment on admission helps us to look carefully for high-risk factors previously undetected or new factors that have since appeared.

The process of birth is the most dangerous journey any individual undertakes.

On admission to the labour ward the history is summarized taking particular note of high-risk factors such as previous perinatal loss, previous or existing intrauterine growth restriction (retardation), bleeding in pregnancy, diabetes mellitus, reduced fetal movements and a variety of other markers. Breech presentation and multiple pregnancy are obvious high-risk factors. On examination general features such as height, weight, blood pressure, temperature and signs of anaemia are reviewed. Before proceeding to vaginal examination, abdominal examination must be complete. This includes a measurement of abdominal size, an estimate of fetal size, lie, presentation and station of the presenting part. The nature of the contractions, amniotic fluid volume estimation and auscultation of the fetal heart complete this procedure. Traditionally the size of the abdomen and fetus is assessed subjectively. The value of formalizing this with an objective value has been suggested in recent years.[3] A measure of the fundosymphysis height (FSH) in centimetres (Figures 2.1 and 2.2) provides a reliable guide to fetal size so long as the observers have been trained in the technique.[4,5] The fundus should not be actively pushed down during the palpation. Ideally a blinded measurement using the blank side of a tape measure is

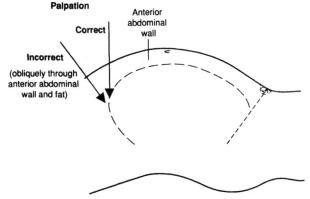

Figure 2.1   Detecting the fundus for fundosymphysis height (FSH) measurement

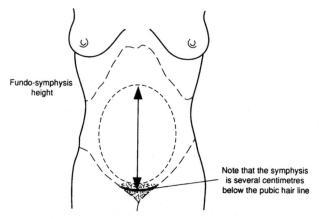

Figure 2.2   Measurement of FSH

desirable. Due attention should be paid to the possible confounding factors of obesity, polyhydramnios, fibroids or unusual physical characteristics of the mother. After 20 weeks' gestation the FSH should be equivalent to the gestational age in centimetres ±2 cm up to 36 weeks, ±3 cm after 36 weeks. No test should be subjected to unrealistic expectations. A tape measure is cheap, available and reasonably reliable with little inter- or intra-observer variation.[6] We are not good at identifying small babies *in utero*; this is obvious from studies of adverse perinatal outcome. The reduced fundosymphysis height may contain a small fetus who may be suffering from chronic asphyxia (intrauterine growth restriction, see Chapter 6). Such a fetus is more likely to develop an abnormal heart rate pattern. A suspicion of a large fetus is also important so that we can anticipate and prepare for mechanical problems. A history of big babies, shoulder dystocia and diabetes mellitus are all important indicators. A rewarding exercise is recording the estimated fetal weight on the partogram. With experience and regular practice this becomes reliable. Management may be altered if abnormal labour progress becomes manifest and there is a likelihood of cephalopelvic disproportion. Marking 'Beware shoulder dystocia' in the 'special features' box on the partogram of women carrying large babies and especially with a history of shoulder dystocia is an important preventative measure. Medical help will be organized to be readily available in the second stage of labour.

Abdominal examination is performed before vaginal examination.

Vaginal examination is undertaken after abdominal palpation. Progressive changes in the uterine cervix permit a diagnosis of labour to be made in the presence of painful uterine contractions occurring at least once every 10 minutes with or without a show or spontaneous rupture of the membranes. This is an important diagnosis. Without it the mother will not be kept in the labour ward with the likelihood of ill-advised intervention. In this situation the best decision is often to do nothing rather than to do something. Inexperienced medical staff seem sometimes to feel an irrational pressure to intervene. If there has been spontaneous rupture of the membranes without labour being present (prelabour rupture of the membranes) then digital examination should not be performed unless a decision has already been taken to proceed to delivery. Umbilical cord compression can be excluded by running a strip of fetal heart rate tracing without recourse to digital examination. The colour of the amniotic fluid should be recorded.

In all cases, whether labour is becoming established or not, an admission cardiotocographic tracing (CTG) – admission test – should be performed. The principle of the admission test and its scientific justification will be explained in detail in Chapter 7. After this clinical review a decision can be taken about the application of appropriate technology for the rest of the labour. This may consist of mobilization and intermittent monitoring (low risk), continuous electronic monitoring (high risk) or most commonly a sequential combination of both. Full information should be provided to the woman and her wishes carefully considered. It should be emphasized that in every case when electronic monitoring is not being

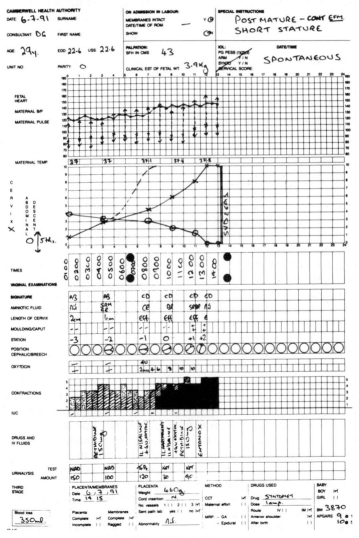

Figure 2.3   Partogram (King's College Hospital)

performed then skilled, careful intermittent auscultation is undertaken.

All observations are then plotted on a partogram as shown in Figure 2.3. These should be tailored to the individual case. Maternal temperature should be checked 4-hourly when the previous recording has been normal. Pulse rate and blood pressure are recorded every hour when the previous observations have been normal with no protein detected in the urine. Abdominal palpation is recorded every 4 hours prior to a vaginal examination. Urine is tested for ketones, protein and glucose whenever it is produced. The programme of observations should not be rigid and will vary depending on the clinical situation.

The admission assessment is particularly important with a view to undertaking safe intermittent, limited electronic monitoring. The mother's degree of risk may change from low to high; however, indications will usually be present. A normal admission CTG in a mother who, on history and examination, is low risk assures a healthy fetus for the next 4 hours unless one of four events supervenes:

1 placental abruption
2 umbilical cord prolapse
3 injudicious use of oxytocics
4 imprudent application of instruments.

Placental abruption is characterized by pain, anxiety, tachycardia and often bleeding; a good midwife or doctor should suspect and detect it. Umbilical cord prolapse occurs after rupture of the membranes with a high presenting part. Good midwifery and medical practice should detect this early when it occurs in the labour ward and the outcome for this condition is excellent when properly treated. The proper use of oxytocics and appropriate electronic monitoring (see Chapter 10) and the proper use of instruments are promoted by education and training. Death of a normally formed term fetus within 4 hours of a normal CTG is a rare event but certainly can occur with a serious placental abruption for which there may be no warning sign. A fetus can die of placental abruption within 15 minutes of a normal CTG.

The importance of clinical sense cannot be overemphasized. Figure 2.4 shows the 'complete' CTG machine including an accompanying tape measure and fetal stethoscope. Why the fetal stethoscope? The CTG shown in Figure 2.5 was undertaken in a mother admitted complaining of reduced fetal movements. The fetal stethoscope was not used and the ultrasound transducer applied directly to the maternal abdomen. The mother was reassured that the baby was healthy; however a macerated stillbirth occurred 1

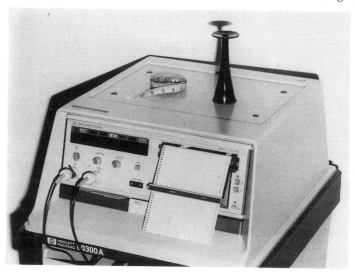

Figure 2.4 'Complete' fetal monitor

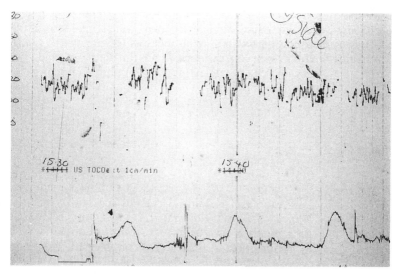

Figure 2.5 'CTG' of dead baby – ultrasound

hour later. The heart rate picked up was maternal pulse from a major vessel with the ultrasound beam having passed through the dead fetus. The mother had a tachycardia on account of her anxiety. Figure 2.6 is the trace obtained when the mother was admitted draining thick meconium and a scalp electrode was applied with

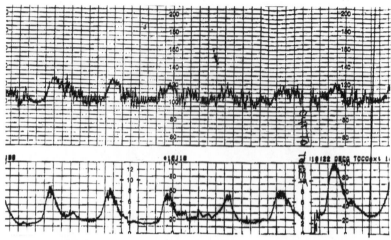

Figure 2.6   'CTG' of dead baby – fetal electrode

some urgency. The midwives were reassured by the trace but the baby was born shortly thereafter as a macerated stillbirth. It was growth restricted and had died of hypoxia some time before. On account of oligohydramnios the fetal buttocks were in contact with the fundus which in turn was in contact with the diaphragm and the path of transmission of the maternal ECG through the fetus is clear.

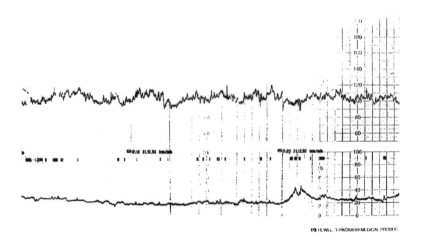

Figure 2.7   'CTG' of dead baby – ultrasound with fetal movement profile

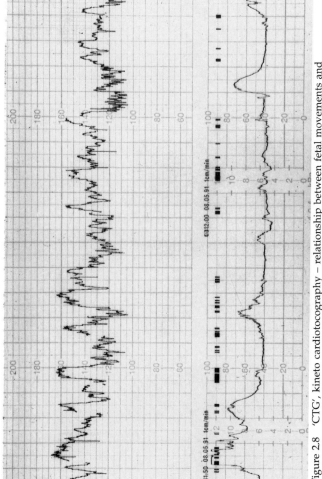

Figure 2.8 'CTG', kineto cardiotocography – relationship between fetal movements and accelerations of FHR

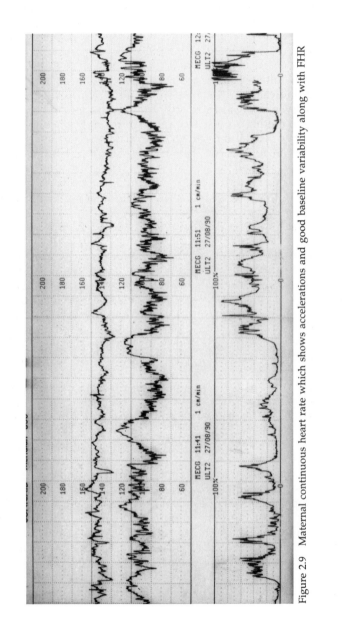

Figure 2.9 Maternal continuous heart rate which shows accelerations and good baseline variability along with FHR

The scalp electrode therefore may capture the maternal ECG when the fetus is dead. The stethoscope must always be used to establish a fetal pulse different from the maternal pulse. Figure 2.7 is the trace obtained when the mother attended not in labour but complaining of reduced fetal movements. The midwives applied the Hewlett Packard 1350 fetal monitor which includes a fetal movement detector in the ultrasound transducer. The black lines in the middle of the trace indicate movements. The mother returned some hours later and delivered a macerated stillbirth. The ultrasound had again picked up the mother's pulse but, more worryingly, the movements detected were not fetal movements but maternal intestinal activity or other maternal movement. It should be noted that adult heart rate recordings also show baseline variability and accelerations. Proper clinical application should help us to avoid these tragic pitfalls. The mother's pulse rate should be correlated to the fetal heart rate and annotated at the beginning of the trace.

Figure 2.8 shows the correct use of the 'kineto cardiotocograph' on the Hewlett Packard 1350 monitor showing the physiological truth of the relationship between true fetal movements and acceleration of the fetal heart. Figure 2.9 shows the correct use of maternal continuous heart rate recording as now available on all intrapartum fetal monitors, demonstrating clearly that, not surprisingly, the adult heart shows accelerations and baseline variability. Understanding this should reduce confusion in distinguishing one heart rate from the other. The use of such a facility is ideally suited but much underused in the scenario of managing preterm labour with beta sympathomimetic therapy.

The importance of clinical sense cannot be overemphasized.

Incidentally Figure 2.5 also shows a common day-to-day error: the incorrect setting of the clock mechanism recording the time on the trace. This may be user error, particularly frequent after a seasonal time change, or the batteries in the machine may be running low. It should be very simply corrected.

Good communication with the mother and her partner is vital. Obstetric cases are unique in that they are not sick, as are patients in all other departments of the hospital. On the contrary, they are experiencing one of the most important events in their lives with enormous emotional impact. The intimacy of this should not be compromised except in the 'genuine interest' of safety for mother and child. This book should help us to recognize this 'genuine interest'. Without this we will not earn the approbation of those who have entrusted their care to us.

Chapter 3

Electronic fetal monitoring: terminology

Even when we all speak one language there remain difficulties in communication because of differing use of terminology. This may be resolved by better understanding and consideration of terms and definitions agreed by the International Federation of Obstetrics and Gynaecology (FIGO) Subcommittee on Standards in Perinatal Medicine. These recommendations were published in 1987 in the *International Journal of Gynecology and Obstetrics*[7] and are largely used in this text. Without a consistency of terminology we cannot have a consistency of interpretation.

Monitoring is first of all clinical and then complemented by technological methods. No cardiotocograph (CTG) can be interpreted without careful appraisal of the clinical situation. The following list illustrates particularly high-risk factors: prematurity, postmaturity, poor fetal growth, reduced fetal movements, meconium-stained amniotic fluid, bleeding in pregnancy, high blood pressure, breech presentation, multiple pregnancy and diabetes mellitus. This list could be extended indefinitely and yet would still only account for a minority of women delivering babies in most labour wards. Recognition of these factors is critical.

In the UK we refer to antepartum CTGs and intrapartum CTGs. In the USA antepartum CTGs are referred to as non-stress tests (NSTs). These are therefore distinguished from contraction stress tests (CSTs) where the contractions are stimulated by exogenous oxytocin. In the UK, CSTs are not performed and reliance is placed on other biophysical tests of fetal well-being. The admission test is a natural contraction stress test using the contractions of early labour.

A fetal heart rate tracing should be technically adequate to warrant analysis. The pen heat should not be too high because it can produce a very dark trace, occasionally burning the paper, or too low, producing a faint trace. This can be adjusted on most machines; however, it is also affected by using the incorrect paper for that machine. The length of the CTG strip depends on the paper speed. In the UK it is usually 1 cm/minute while in the USA it is 3 cm/minute. As the pattern of the trace is dramatically altered by a change in paper speed, this can lead to confusion. It should, therefore, be standardized. Because there is not much to be gained by the faster paper speed with a consequent greater consumption of paper, the slower speed of 1 cm/minute should be selected. Each vertical division on the paper is 1 cm and therefore 1 minute. A tracing should be annotated fully. At the beginning of the trace the mother's name, reference number and pulse rate should be recorded. Modern machines automatically annotate the time and date; however, a human being has to ensure that they are correctly set in the software and changed as the clock time changes, notably with the onset of 'summer time'. The newest monitors have keypads or bar-code readers with which any other information may be recorded on the trace. This is important to relate vaginal examination, change of posture, epidural and other transient events to the fetal heart rate pattern, which could have medico-legal implications at a later date. The vertical scale on the paper should be standardized to display between 50 and 210 beats per minute in order for visual perception and interpretation to be consistent.

A tracing should be annotated fully.

The *baseline fetal heart rate* is the mean level of the fetal heart rate when this is stable with accelerations and decelerations excluded. It is determined over a time period of 5 or 10 minutes and expressed in beats per minute (bpm). The rate may gradually change over time; however, for one particular period it normally remains fairly constant. Contrary to traditional teaching the normal range of the

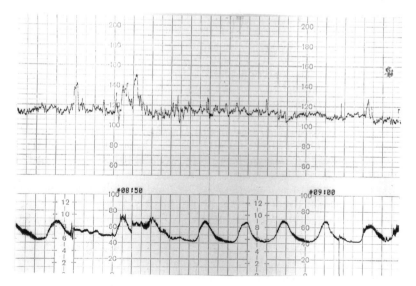

Figure 3.1 CTG: baseline fetal heart rate of 112 bpm

baseline fetal heart rate at term is 110–150 bpm.[7,8] Previously rates between 110 and 120 bpm have been classified as mild baseline bradycardia. Close involvement in the labour ward shows us that this is a relatively frequent finding. Providing the baseline rate is steady and not declining and that there are accelerations with normal variability, the outcome is excellent (Figure 3.1). However, fetuses at term with a baseline heart rate of between 150 and 160 bpm cannot be regarded in the same way. Such a situation occurs in the late first stage and second stage of a prolonged labour when the mother is tired, dehydrated and ketotic (Figure 3.2a). If corrective measures are not undertaken the rate will rise to 160 and 170 bpm (Figure 3.2b). This represents progressive asphyxia and is not an ideal scenario for a difficult instrumental vaginal delivery. Asphyxia is more likely to develop with a baseline rate of 155 compared to ll5 bpm. This statement must be qualified before 34 weeks' gestation when the baseline fetal heart rate tends to be higher and a rate of up to 160 bpm is acceptable. Difficulty in identifying the baseline is considered in Chapter 5.

A *bradycardia* is a baseline heart rate of less than 110 bpm. A rate of 100–110 bpm is termed moderate baseline bradycardia. Provided there are accelerations, good baseline variability and no decelerations this is considered normal and associated with a healthy fetus. Hypoxia should be suspected if a rate is below 100 bpm.

A *tachycardia* is a baseline heart rate of more than 150 bpm. If the baseline rate is between 150 and 170 bpm it is termed moderate baseline tachycardia and provided other features are reassuring it is associated with a healthy fetus.

An *acceleration* is defined as a transient increase in heart rate of 15 bpm or more and lasting 15 seconds or more. The recording of at least two accelerations in a 20-minute period is considered a *reactive trace*. Accelerations are considered a good sign of fetal health: the fetus is responding to stimuli and displaying integrity of its mechanisms controlling the fetal heart. Accelerations may merge or be continuous suggesting a tachycardia. As explained later, comprehensive analysis of the clinical situation with a very active fetus may clarify this.

A *deceleration* is a transient episode of slowing of the fetal heart rate below the baseline level of more than 15 bpm and lasting 15 seconds or more. Decelerations may be greater than this but not significant when other features of the heart rate are normal. The WHO/FIGO definition of duration of a deceleration is 10 seconds which is too short and includes many normal patterns. When there is an abnormal variability (less than 5 bpm) in a non-reactive trace, decelerations may be very significant even when less than 15 bpm in amplitude (see later). A deceleration immediately following an acceleration recovering within 30 seconds is considered normal.

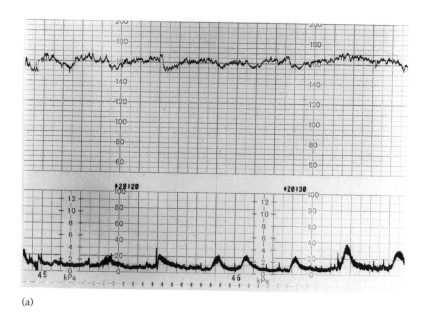

(a)

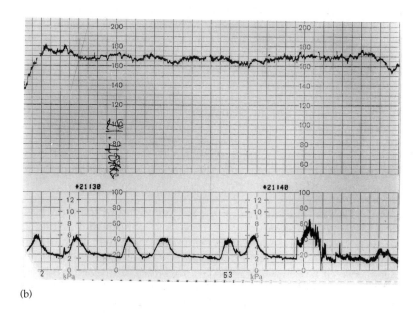

(b)

Figure 3.2 (a) Baseline rate 155–160 bpm; (b) rising to 165–170 bpm

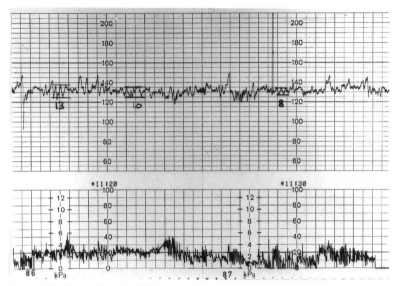

Figure 3.3   Normal band width

Baseline variability is the degree to which the baseline varies within a particular *band width* excluding accelerations and decelerations (Figure 3.3). This is a function of the oscillatory amplitude of the baseline. For the purposes of research projects oscillatory frequency and oscillatory amplitude may be quantified and scored. This is too complex for routine clinical use and band width is preferred. Figure 3.4 shows band widths classified as silent pattern (0–5), reduced (5–10), normal (10–25) and saltatory (more than 25). The baseline variability indicates the integrity of the autonomic nervous system. It should be assessed during a reactive period in a 1-minute segment showing the greatest band width. Strictly speaking beat-to-beat variation is not seen on traces. The equipment is not designed to analyse every beat interval and uses an averaging technique. In a 1-minute interval one cannot see 140 discrete dots. In a research situation beat-to-beat variation can be analysed and is proportionally related to baseline variability. Some workers classify beat-to-beat variation as short-term variability and baseline variability as long-term variability. An understanding of the mechanism of production of baseline variability is crucial to an understanding of fetal heart rate interpretation (see Chapter 4).

Decelerations are *early, late* or *variable*. Early decelerations are synchronous with contractions, are usually associated with fetal head compression and therefore appear in the late first stage and second stage of labour with descent of the head. They are usually,

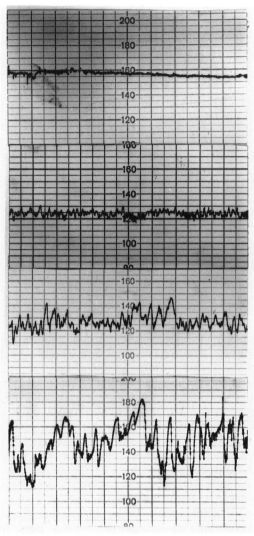

Figure 3.4   Band width classification (reading downwards): silent, 0–5 bpm; reduced, 6–10 bpm; normal, 11–25 bpm; saltatory, over 25 bpm

but not invariably, benign. Late decelerations are exactly what their name implies with respect to the contractions. As shown in Figure 3.5 the onset, nadir and recovery are all out of phase with the contraction. They are usually, but not invariably, pathological. The use of the terminology of type I and type II dips does not contribute to further understanding. Variable decelerations vary in shape and

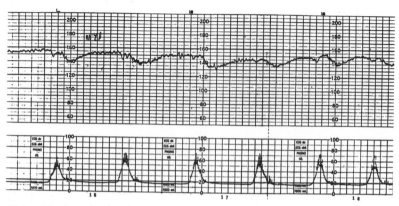

Figure 3.5   Late deceleration

sometimes in timing with respect to each other. They may or may not indicate hypoxia. Misconceptions have been perpetuated for many years about the need to categorize exactly decelerations in these groups. Much valuable time has been wasted in fruitless discussions about this classification of timing. What is critical is the fetal condition between decelerations and its evolution with time. The integrity of the autonomic control system of the fetal heart must be evaluated (see Chapter 4).

Fetal distress, as implied from a CTG appearance, is not always indicative of hypoxia. Many fetuses are stressed and the challenge is to recognize when this progresses to hypoxic distress. Many babies are delivered operatively for fetal distress (abnormal CTG) and are in excellent condition. This is the crux of the matter in considering the increased caesarean section rate after the introduction of electronic fetal monitoring. We do not *see* fetal distress on a strip of CTG paper. We *see* a fetal heart rate pattern and should describe and classify it as such. It should then be interpreted with respect to the probability of it representing fetal compromise. Anaemia (a low haemoglobin concentration) is not treated rationally without further consideration being given to its aetiology. The same should apply to a fetal heart rate pattern that is not normal. In the light of the clinical situation the likelihood of hypoxia and/or acidosis can be evaluated.

Chapter 4

Control of the fetal heart

Control of the fetal heart is complex (Figure 4.1). The fetal heart has its own intrinsic activity and a rate determined by the spontaneous activity of the pacemaker in the sinoatrial node; this structure has the fastest rate and determines the rate in the normal heart. The next fastest pacemaker is in the atrium. The atrioventricular node has the slowest rate of activity and generates the idioventricular rhythm seen in complete heart block. Under the circumstances of complete heart block the ventricle beats at 60–80 bpm.

The fetal heart rate is modulated by a number of stimuli. Central nervous system influence is important with cortical and subcortical influences not under voluntary control. We cannot alter our heart rate at will. The cardioregulatory centre in the brainstem also plays a part. Other physiological factors regulate the heart rate such as circulatory catecholamines, chemoreceptors, baroreceptors and their interplay with the autonomic nervous system.[9]

The efferent component of the autonomic nervous system is composed of the sympathetic and parasympathetic systems. There is a constant input from these systems varying from second to second. Sympathetic impulses drive the heart rate to increase while parasympathetic impulses have the opposite effect. If we are confronted with a frightening situation our heart rate involuntarily increases. This puts us under stress, sometimes distress; however, it is an adaptive mechanism preparing us for fright or flight – the sympathetic response. On the contrary, if we are feeling very relaxed and happy at home in the evening after a busy day our heart rate will decrease on account of parasympathetic stimulation.

Electronic fetal heart rate monitors compute the heart rate based on averaged intervals between beats extrapolated to what the rate would if that beat interval remained constant. The machine produces a rate read out after only being applied for a few seconds. However, autonomic impulses immediately and constantly take effect changing the beat intervals and immediately altering the heart rate. This is how baseline variability is generated and it indicates integrity of the autonomic nervous system (Figure 4.2). Baseline variability is actually seen on the tracing. If it is greatly magnified

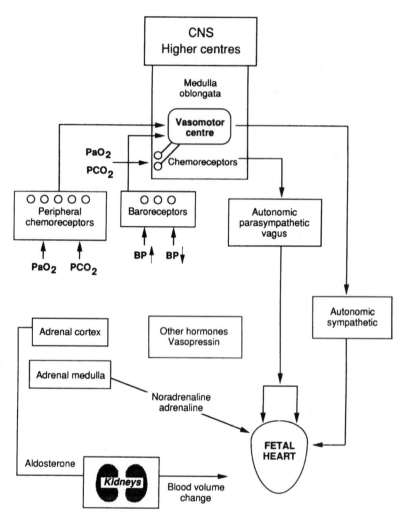

Figure 4.1   Control of the fetal heart. CNS, central nervous system; BP, blood pressure

individual beats, beat-to-beat variation, can be seen with special equipment used for physiological studies (Figure 4.3). In practice, baseline variability is the preferred term. The sympathetic nervous system plays a similar role in the genesis of accelerations. In addition, the parasympathetic or vagal system has a specific effect of generating baseline variability. Suppression of vagal impulses by a drug such as atropine reduces baseline variability. Physiological mechanisms are complex and incompletely understood. Fortunately

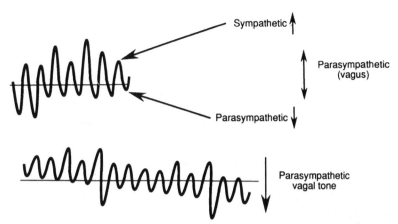

Figure 4.2 Baseline variability: autonomic modulation

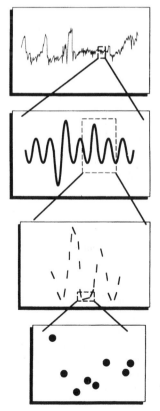

Figure 4.3 Baseline variability: beat-to-beat variation

the autonomic nervous system is sensitive to hypoxia at a critical level for the fetus and changes in this response are therefore used as important indicators of well-being. The sympathetic and parasympathetic systems mature at slightly different rates with respect to gestational age. The sympathetic system matures faster and this results in marginally faster baseline rates in the preterm period. It is of some interest that boy fetuses have slightly faster heart rates than girl fetuses; however, this is of absolutely no diagnostic value. Before 34 weeks of gestation a higher baseline rate is to be expected. Accelerations and normal baseline variability suggest good autonomic control and therefore little likelihood of hypoxia.

Pathophysiological mechanisms of decelerations

An understanding of the maintenance of autonomic control and the mechanisms of decelerations is important. The following illustrations show the effects of contractions on the fetus and blood flow in diagrammatic form (Figure 4.4).

Early decelerations are early in timing with respect to the uterine contractions and this is therefore a better term than type I dips. They are most commonly due to compression of the fetal head. A rise in intracranial pressure is associated with stimulation of the vagal nerve and bradycardia. This may be caused by a uterine contraction and the sequence of events in this situation is shown in Figures 4.5–4.9. Head compression decelerations are most frequently seen in the late stages of labour when descent of the head is occurring. Indeed, on some occasions the onset of the second stage of labour can be deduced from the tracing. Decelerations due to head compression are seen at the time of vaginal examination and also when artificial rupture of the membranes has been performed. Early

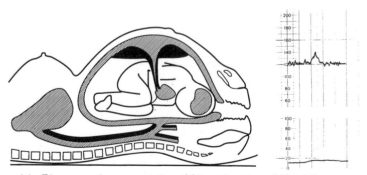

Figure 4.4   Diagrammatic representation of fetus, placenta and blood flow

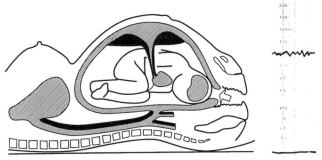

Figure 4.5   Early deceleration: start of contraction

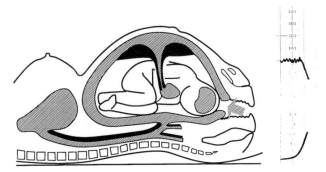

Figure 4.6   Early deceleration: increasing contraction

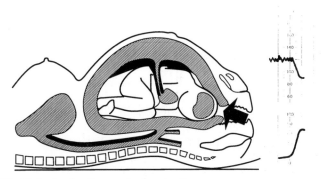

Figure 4.7   Early deceleration: peak of contraction

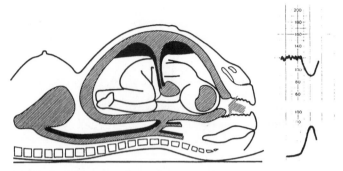

Figure 4.8   Early deceleration: decreasing contraction

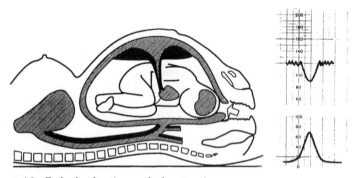

Figure 4.9   Early deceleration: end of contraction

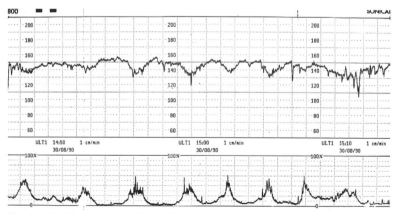

Figure 4.10   Example of early decelerations

decelerations with contractions are symmetrical and bell-shaped (Figure 4.10). The clinical situation should be reviewed to ensure that head compression is a likely explanation at that time. If not, and if the trace is atypical, then an apparently innocuous early deceleration may be pathological. In one case the obstetric registrar reported that a young West Indian nullipara suffering from sickle cell disease at term but with abdominal size and scan suggesting intrauterine growth restriction was 'niggling' but not yet in established labour. The fetal head was unengaged. He reported the trace (Figure 4.11) as showing early decelerations. He wished to proceed to induction of labour but the consultant suggested he proceed directly to caesarean section. The registrar was surprised but learned an important lesson on delivering a significantly growth restricted baby covered in meconium with Apgar scores of 5 and 6 who made a satisfactory recovery. Review of the trace the following day showed that although the decelerations might be described by some as early they do show poor recovery of the second one, no accelerations and a suggestion of reduced variability after the second deceleration. What is more important is that this fetus had no reason to have head compression and also had a background of risk.

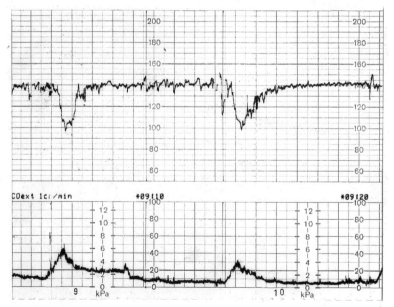

Figure 4.11   Pathological 'early' deceleration (more likely to be variable) – head 4/5 to 5/5 palpable

Late decelerations are late in timing with respect to the uterine contraction and are therefore best described as such rather than as type II dips. The suggested pathophysiological mechanism of such decelerations is shown in Figures 4.12–4.14. There is a reservoir of

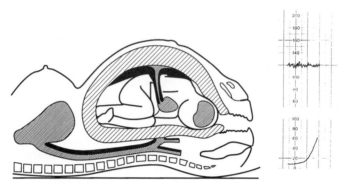

Figure 4.12   Late deceleration: start of contraction

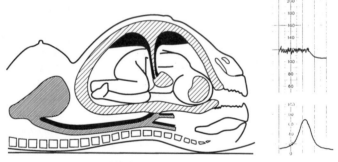

Figure 4.13   Late deceleration: after peak of contraction

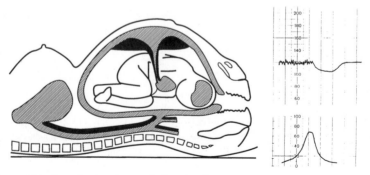

Figure 4.14   Late deceleration: end of contraction

oxygenated blood in the retroplacental space. The size of this space varies and is smaller in intrauterine growth restriction. Poor blood flow to the uteroplacental space is characteristic of fetuses with intrauterine growth restriction. As a contraction begins the fetus uses up the reservoir of oxygen in the retroplacental space. Due to the restricted supply of blood a hypoxic deceleration begins, it continues through the contraction and does not recover fully until some time after the contraction, when full oxygenation has been restored. The speed of recovery on the ascending limb may reflect the blood flow and the resilience of the fetus. In a non-hypoxic fetus there is increased variability during a deceleration on account of autonomic response. When hypoxia develops there is a tendency to reduced variability.

Baseline variability and decelerations – exception to the rule

A deceleration is defined when the fetal heart rate decelerates by more than 15 beats from the baseline for more than 15 seconds. However, this rule does not apply when the baseline variability is less than 5 beats and any deceleration, even less than 15 beats from the baseline, could be ominous (Figure 4.15) unless otherwise proven.

Variable decelerations hold the key to understanding fetal heart rate patterns and are the most common of all. They are called variable because they vary in shape, size and sometimes in timing with

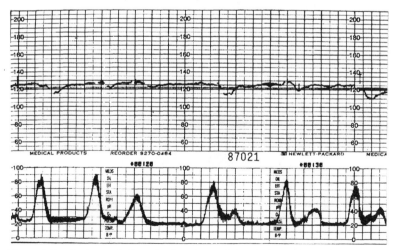

Figure 4.15   Ominous shallow deceleration with baseline variability <5 bpm

respect to each other. They vary because they are a manifestation of compression of the umbilical cord and it is compressed in a slightly different way each time. On some occasions it may not be compressed at all and there is no deceleration with that particular contraction. Variable decelerations are more often seen when the amniotic fluid volume is reduced. In North America they are referred to as cord compression decelerations.

The mechanism is illustrated in Figures 4.16–4.20. The umbilical vein has a thinner wall and lower intraluminal pressure than the umbilical arteries (Figure 4.16). When compression occurs the blood flow through the vein is interrupted before that through the artery. The fetus therefore loses some of its circulating blood volume. When a healthy individual or fetus loses some of its circulating blood

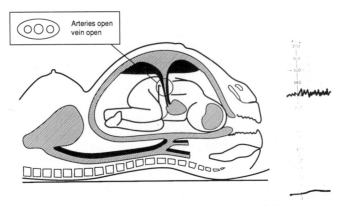

Figure 4.16 Umbilical cord, fetus and placenta: normal circulation

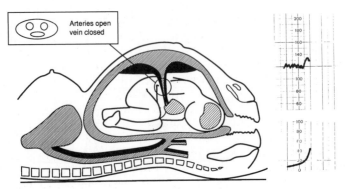

Figure 4.17 Variable deceleration: start of contraction

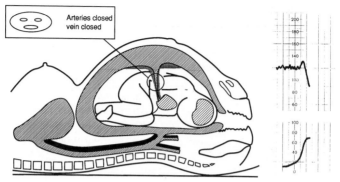

Figure 4.18   Variable deceleration: increasing contraction

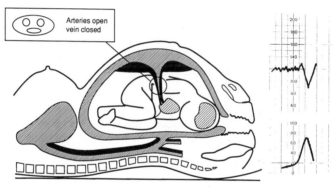

Figure 4.19   Variable deceleration: decreasing contraction

volume the natural response effected by the autonomic nervous system is a rise in pulse rate to compensate. A small acceleration therefore appears at the start of a variable deceleration when the fetus is not compromised (Figure 4.17). After that the umbilical arteries are also occluded, the circulation is relatively restored followed by an increase in systemic pressure, the baroreceptors are stimulated and there is a precipitous fall in the fetal heart rate (Figure 4.18). The deceleration is at its nadir with both vessels occluded. During release of the cord compression arterial flow is restored first with a consequent autonomically mediated sharp rise in heart rate (Figure 4.19) due to systemic hypotension of blood being pumped out culminating in a small acceleration after the deceleration (Figure 4.20). These accelerations before and after decelerations are called *shouldering*. Whatever they are called, they are a manifestation of a fetus coping well with cord compression.

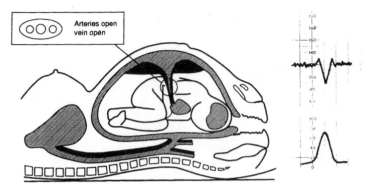

Figure 4.20   Variable deceleration: end of contraction

The way the cord is being compressed will vary depending exactly on how it is positioned with respect to the structure compressing it. On the same basis, variable decelerations may change if the posture of the mother is changed. Normal well-grown fetuses can tolerate cord compression for a considerable length of time before they become hypoxic. Small growth-restricted fetuses do not have the same resilience. To assess this process it is necessary to analyse the features of the decelerations and also the character of the trace as it evolves. Figure 4.21 shows:

1 normal shouldering
2 exaggeration of shouldering or overshoot which is thought to be prepathological
3 loss of shouldering–pathological
4 smoothing of the baseline variability within the deceleration which is associated with loss of variability at the baseline and therefore pathological
5 late recovery – having the same pathological significance as late deceleration
6 biphasic deceleration requiring the same consideration as a late deceleration

If the duration of the deceleration is more than 60 seconds and the depth greater than 60 beats, progressive hypoxia becomes more likely.

The most critical feature, however, is the evolution of the trace with time. A change in the baseline rate and change in the baseline variability are the key signs of developing hypoxia and acidosis. Figure 4.22 shows two strips of CTG 60 minutes apart. In spite of marked variable decelerations, the baseline rate and baseline

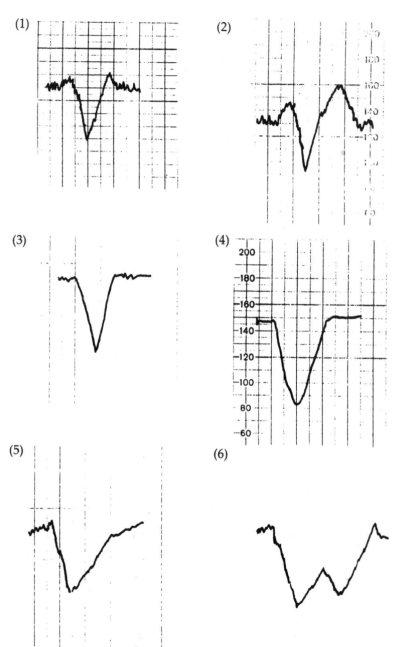

Figure 4.21   Features of variable decelerations

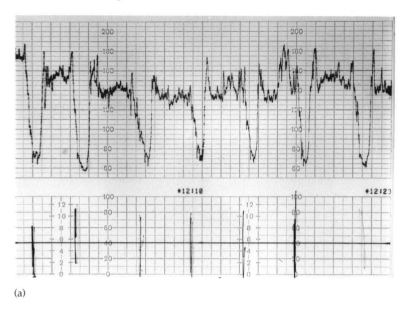

(a)

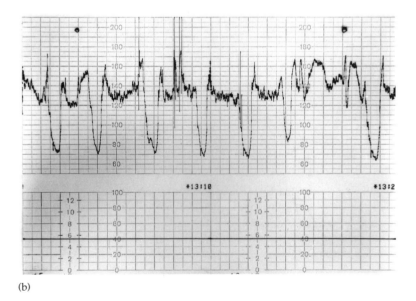

(b)

Figure 4.22   Two CTGs recorded 60 minutes apart, showing variable decelerations without abnormal features (suspicious trace)

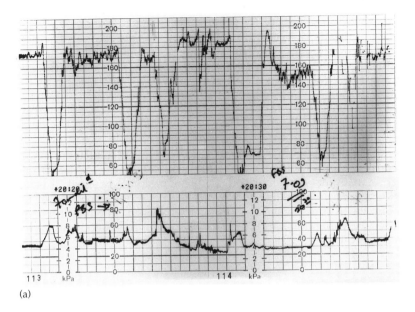

(a)

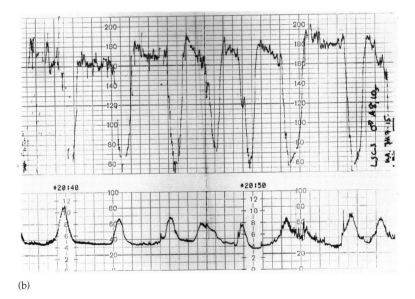

(b)

Figure 4.23   Two CTGs recorded 20 minutes apart. (a) Variable decelerations with abnormal features (duration >60 seconds, depth >60 beats; tachycardia) (abnormal trace); (b) suggestive of distress (tachycardia and reduced baseline variability)

variability are maintained. So long as adequate progress is being made towards delivery this trace need not cause concern. Figure 4.23 also shows two strips of trace 20 minutes apart but with quite different features. The progression to a tachycardia with reduced variability suggests developing hypoxia. The time required for a fetus with a previously normal trace to become acidotic related to different patterns of the fetal heart rate has been studied.[10] In many cases it will take over 100 minutes. Medical staff should have time enough to identify the problem and act effectively.

Much time is wasted in discussion over whether decelerations are early, late or variable and whether they can be pigeon-holed into good, bad and possibly good. Such discussion is fruitless. It is not the deceleration itself that is critical but it is the evolution of the trace with time. The baseline rate between decelerations, the baseline variability and the presence or absence of accelerations are critical.

Classification of fetal heart rate pattern

The FIGO subcommittee proposed the useful classification of CTG as: (a) normal, (b) suspicious and (c) pathological.

Intrapartum

Normal pattern

1 Baseline rate between 110 and 150 bpm.
2 Amplitude of heart rate variability between 5 and 25 bpm. (FIGO do not refer to accelerations but they should be present.)

Suspicious pattern

1 Baseline heart rate between 150 and 170 bpm or between 110 and 100 bpm.
2 Amplitude of variability between 5 and 10 bpm for more than 40 minutes.
3 Increased variability above 25 bpm.
4 Variable decelerations.

Pathological pattern

1 Baseline heart rate below 100 bpm or above 170 bpm.
2 Persistence of heart rate variability of less than 5 bpm for more than 40 minutes.

3 Severe variable decelerations or severe repetitive early decelerations.
4 Prolonged decelerations.
5 Late decelerations: the most *ominous* trace is a steady baseline without baseline variability and with small decelerations after each contraction.
6 Sinusoidal pattern is regular with cyclic changes in the fetal heart rate baseline such as the sine wave. The characteristics of the pattern being: the frequency is less than 6 cycles per minute, the amplitude is at least 10 bpm and the duration should be 20 minutes or longer.

Normal implies that the trace assures fetal health. Suspicious indicates that continued observation or additional simple tests are required to ensure fetal health. Pathological, better described as abnormal, warrants some action in the form of additional tests or delivery depending on the clinical picture. Abnormal may not be pathological in the true sense of the word.

The expression fetal distress should be reconsidered. A trace that is not normal may result from physiological, iatrogenic or pathological causes. The clinical situation and the dynamic evolution of features of the trace with time will clarify the situation.

The underlying principle is to detect fetal compromise using the concept of 'fetal distress' very critically. In all situations, it is consideration of the overall clinical picture that will provide the clues as to whether fetal compromise is present. Many suspicious CTGs are generated by healthy fetuses demonstrating the ability to respond to stress. For the purposes of clinical decision, scoring systems or computer analysis have not been found to be useful, particularly in the intrapartum period.

Chapter 5

Cardiotocographic interpretation: the basics

A fetal heart rate (FHR) trace has four easily definable features: baseline rate, baseline variability, accelerations and decelerations. The baseline rate (normal 110–150 bpm) is identified by drawing a line through the midpoint of the 'wiggliness' which represents the most common rate having excluded accelerations and decelerations. The baseline variability (normal 10–25 bpm) is determined by drawing horizontal lines at the level of the highest point of the peak and lowest point of the troughs of the 'wiggliness' of the trace in a 1-cm segment (Figure 5.1).

The dynamic state of the fetal cardiovascular system and the concept of fetal behavioural state must be appreciated. Fetuses are recognized as having quiet periods associated with rapid eye movements and active periods without such movements. Active movements are associated with good variability and accelerations. Quiet sleep is associated with episodes of decreased variability

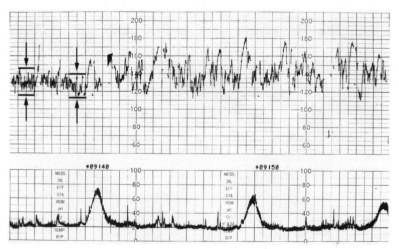

Figure 5.1 'Wiggliness' of the baseline – determination of baseline variability (best segment representative of autonomic nervous system activity to be chosen)

which generally last for up to 40 minutes. Interpretation of a trace is absolutely dependent on recognition of this physiological phenomenon. Baseline variability is best interpreted during the active phase, recognized by the presence of accelerations defined as rises of 15 beats or more lasting for 15 seconds or more. The presence of two accelerations in a 20-minute trace is termed a reactive trace and is suggestive of a fetus in good health. These fetuses usually have normal variability. A trace can be described as reactive within a short time once a normal baseline rate, normal baseline variability and accelerations are identified. However, in order to be described as non-reactive it should run for a period of at least 40 minutes during which two accelerations were not identified in any 20-minute period. FHR decelerations describe a transient event. Early decelerations in the late first stage and early second stage of labour generally indicate head compression and rarely compromise. Late decelerations indicate transient hypoxia with impaired uteroplacental perfusion which may well proceed to established acidosis. Variable decelerations are often due to cord compression but are also seen in fetuses in breech presentation and occipitoposterior position when the postulated mechanism is pressure on the supraorbital region of the head. Developing hypoxia and acidosis are suggested

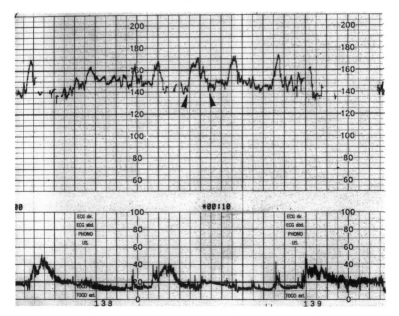

Figure 5.2   Reactive trace – two accelerations in 20 minutes

by the absence of accelerations, a rise in the baseline rate and a reduction in baseline variability.

Accelerations are the hallmark of fetal health

Features of a reactive trace are shown in Figure 5.2. In looking at this trace think of a child playing in a field. The child has a normal pulse rate (baseline rate), minor movements of the limbs suggestive of activity (good baseline variability) and is tossing a ball up and down (accelerations). If the child is tired or is unwell it will start restricting its activity and stop tossing the ball (absence of accelerations is the first thing to be noticed when hypoxia develops) suggesting that either the child is not well or is tired. Then the child would either sit or lie down to rest. In such a situation it is difficult to differentiate healthy tiredness from impending sickness. A persistently raised pulse rate after a period of rest would suggest the latter (baseline tachycardia). The fetus cannot respond to hypoxia by increasing its cardiac stroke volume and has to increase its cardiac output by an increase in heart rate. Reduction in baseline variability and finally a flat baseline are the progressive features with increasing hypoxia. This is analogous to a rapid thready pulse in a sick person and should be borne in mind when analysing traces.

Figure 5.3 shows a reactive trace with accelerations, normal rate, normal variability but a section of the trace was not registered. In the segment after the missing portion there are no accelerations, normal rate but reduced baseline variability. A child who was in good health a few minutes ago cannot suddenly become sick without an obvious

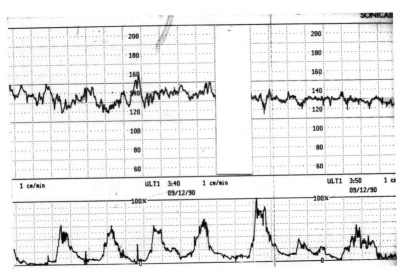

Figure 5.3   Reactive trace with a blank section

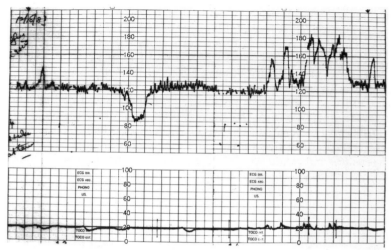

Figure 5.4 Reactive trace with isolated deceleration

reason. The absence of accelerations and reduced baseline variability suggest that the fetus is in the quiet phase. This interpretation is further strengthened because there is no increase in the baseline FHR.

Figure 5.4 shows a trace with baseline FHR of 120 bpm with normal baseline variability and an isolated deceleration followed by marked accelerations. The normal baseline rate and variability with marked accelerations (tossing the ball up and down) suggests that the fetus is not hypoxic. The isolated deceleration may be due to brief cord compression associated with fetal movement. In the intrapartum situation this may be accounted for by fetal movements, uterine contractions or reduced amniotic fluid due to the membranes having ruptured. This is not an immediate threat to the fetus but further continuous electronic fetal monitoring (EFM) is indicated. In the antenatal period the possibility of reduced amniotic fluid has to be considered either due to intrauterine growth restriction, prelabour rupture of the membranes or postmaturity. Ultrasound evaluation should be undertaken. If the amniotic fluid volume is normal the deceleration may be due to pressure on the cord due to fetal movement.

Figure 5.5 shows a trace with repetitive variable decelerations. At the beginning of the trace the baseline rate is 120 bpm, there are no accelerations and the baseline variability is normal. Towards the end of the trace the baseline rate has risen to 160 bpm with decrease in baseline variability. This suggests an attempt to compensate in response to the evolving hypoxia.

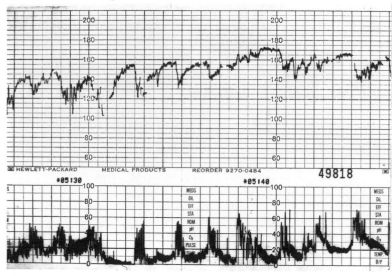

Figure 5.5   Repetitive variable decelerations – developing asphyxia

Paper speed

It is important to check the paper speed of any CTG tracing before interpretation. It is not easy for someone who is trained to interpret traces at 1 cm/minute to interpret a trace recorded at a speed of 3 cm/minute. With current fetal monitoring technology the paper speed is annotated automatically on the trace. If the paper speed is not annotated on the trace, scrutiny of the contraction duration would give a clue that the paper speed is more than 1 cm/minute as the contraction duration on the trace would be 2 to 3 minutes which is an unlikely event in normal labour. Figure 5.6 shows the effect on the trace by changing paper speed during the recording. Figure 5.7 shows comparative traces recorded at different paper speeds. At the faster paper speed (Figure 5.7b) features such as baseline variability, accelerations and decelerations are altered. The baseline variability appears more reduced than actually is the case, accelerations are difficult to identify (Figure 5.7 a and b), and the decelerations appear to be of a longer duration (Figure 5.6). It is the practice in the UK, some European countries and in Asia to use a paper speed of 1 cm/ minute (thus reducing the number of trees being cut down to produce paper), while the practitioners in the USA run the paper at 3 cm/minute. For a trained eye the paper speed does not matter, but for day-to-day interpretation it is better to have the paper speed at the rate the staff is used to – failure to appreciate this has led to

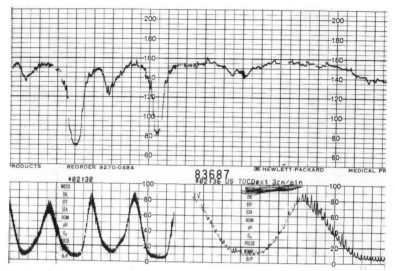

Figure 5.6   Changing paper speed during recording

confusion and serious error. The current fetal monitors have their paper speed switch mechanism either behind the paper loading tray which has to be removed to alter the paper speed (Hewlett Packard 8040) or in a position so that it is difficult to alter the speed accidentally. Although the discussion on paper speed may appear trivial, failure to recognize the difference has resulted in unnecessary caesarean section both in the antenatal and intrapartum period. Such simple mistakes expose the mother to an unnecessary anaesthetic and surgical risk and put her at high risk in her next pregnancy.

Problems associated with the interpretation of the baseline variability

Any FHR tracing has periods of high and low baseline variability cycles both in the antenatal and intrapartum periods. These periods of 'silent phase' with low baseline variability can be as short as 7–10 minutes in the antenatal period[8] and be from 25 to 40 minutes in the intrapartum period.[11] Although baseline variability can be referred to at any given point in the trace, the health of the baby is best judged when the trace is reactive (i.e. when the baby is active and 'playing with the ball' rather than when the baby is sleeping). It is

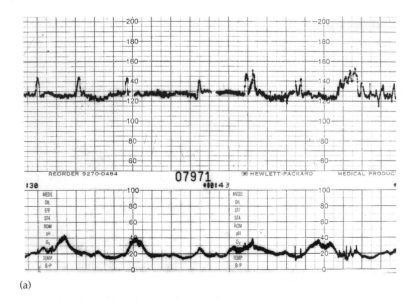

(a)

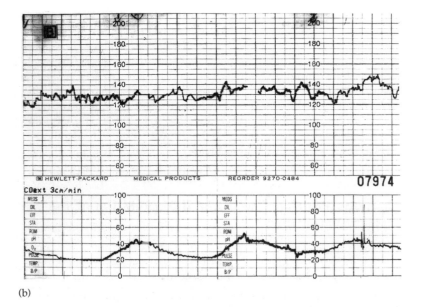

(b)

Figure 5.7   Two recordings from the same patient: (a) at 1 cm/minute, (b) at 3 cm/minute

similar to us being judged at an interview when we are active and awake rather than inactive and sleeping.

Reduced baseline variability

The commonest reasons for reduced baseline variability are:

1 the 'sleep or quiet phase' of the FHR cycle (Figure 5.8)
2 hypoxia
3 prematurity
4 tachycardia
5 drugs (sedatives, antihypertensives acting on the central nervous system, and anaesthetics)
6 local anaesthetic
7 congenital malformation (of the central nervous system more commonly than the cardiovascular system)
8 cardiac arrhythmias
9 fetal anaemia (Rhesus disease or fetomaternal haemorrhage)
10 fetal infection.

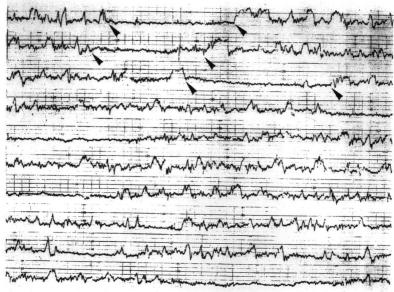

Figure 5.8 Composite trace. Reduced variability: period of fetal 'sleep' alternating with 'active' periods

High and low variability cycles

When a trace is seen with reduced baseline variability (band width <10 bpm), the previous segments of the trace must be reviewed. If the preceding trace was reactive with good baseline variability, then the segment being reviewed is probably in the 'quiet phase' of the baby's FHR cycle and there is no cause for alarm. The start of another active cycle can be awaited especially if there have been no decelerations or increase in the baseline rate which might indicate the possibility of hypoxia. If there was no previous segment of the trace to consider, the clinical picture must be reviewed to identify whether the fetus is at risk (e.g. small fundosymphysis height, post-term, thick meconium, no or scanty amniotic fluid at the time of membrane rupture, reduced fetal movements, other obstetric risk factors) or is influenced by medication (e.g. pethidine, anti-hypertensives etc.) and at the same time continuing the trace when reactivity with good baseline variability may appear.

Pethidine and baseline variability

Sometimes there is concern about giving pethidine to women in labour in case it will reduce the baseline variability and obscure the reduced baseline variability of hypoxia. Before giving pethidine it is important to make sure the FHR trace is reactive and normal with no evidence of hypoxia. Once the pethidine is given, the accelerations may not be evident and the baseline variability may become reduced as in the 'quiet' or 'sleep' phase. The period of this quiet phase following pethidine in some fetuses can extend beyond the natural quiet phase expected and thus leads to anxiety. In labour if the trace has been reactive and the fetus was not hypoxic, hypoxia can develop only gradually due to regular uterine contractions cutting off the blood supply to the placenta, unless acute events such as abruption, cord prolapse, scar dehiscence or oxytocic hyperstimulation occur. Alternatively, it can be due to cord compression with each contraction. The reduction of blood supply to the retroplacental area by regular uterine contractions will present with late decelerations, and hypoxia due to cord compression will present with variable decelerations. If these are affecting the fetus and causing hypoxia, the fetus tends to compensate for the hypoxia by increasing the cardiac output, which it does by increasing the FHR as it has limited capacity to increase the stroke volume. Therefore, if the FHR pattern after pethidine does not show any decelerations and no increase in the baseline rate, despite the fact that there are no accelerations and the baseline variability is reduced, these features are likely to be due to pethidine rather than to hypoxia. When the baby is born, the baby may not cry and may need stimulation or assisted ventilation because of the effect of the drug on the central nervous system causing respiratory depression, but the fetus will have good cord arterial blood status indicating that there was no intrauterine hypoxia.

False baseline variability due to technical reasons

Old machine without autocorrelation

The baseline variability seen on the trace is produced by the time differences between individual heart beats. One segment of the serration or undulation, i.e. one upswing which contributes to baseline variability, is only a few millimetres but is representative of a number of beats, as outlined earlier. The machine calculates the beat intervals from the impulses coming back to the transducer which arise from the movements of the fetal heart. However, there may be extraneous impulses from other sources (caused by movement of bowel or movement of the anterior abdominal wall of the mother) which may be misinterpreted and a falsely exaggerated baseline variability produced (Figure 5.9). When the fetus becomes hypoxic, usually the first feature to be observed is the disappearance of the accelerations, followed by an increase in baseline FHR and a

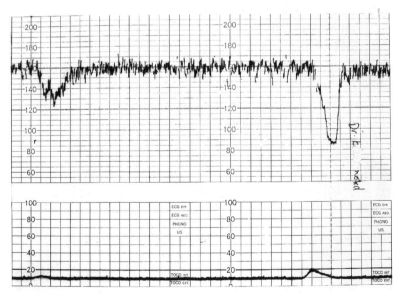

Figure 5.9   Artefactual variability due to an old machine without an autocorrelation facility

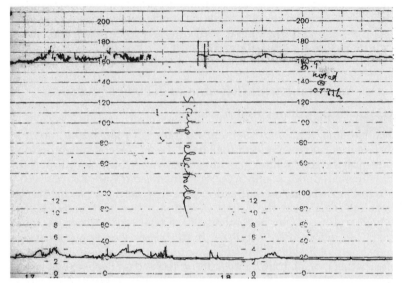

Figure 5.10   Artefactual variability obscuring a pathological trace rectified by using a scalp electrode

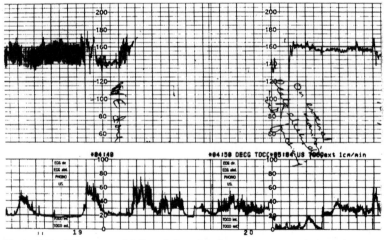

Figure 5.11   Effect on variability of changing the monitoring mode from fetal electrode to ultrasound in a machine with an autocorrelation facility

reduction in the baseline variability. In Figure 5.9, there is tachycardia, with an FHR of 150 bpm, there are no accelerations and there are variable decelerations suggestive of possible fetal compromise. This was from a growth-restricted fetus with little amniotic fluid surrounding it; the other features on the trace (absence of accelerations, tachycardia and decelerations) are not consistent with the 'good baseline variability' observed on the trace. The problem is that the trace was obtained on a fetal monitor without autocorrelation facilities. The baseline variability obtained on the ultrasound mode with the old fetal monitors is not reliable and in labour it is best to use a scalp electrode with these machines. Figure 5.10 shows an abnormal trace with tachycardia, no accelerations and with reduced variability. The switch from ultrasound to direct ECG mode gives the markedly reduced (flat baseline variability) true baseline variability of the sick fetus. Using modern machines should obviate this problem (Figure 5.11).

Poor contact of the scalp electrode

'Picket fence' artefact is not an uncommon problem with the use of scalp electrodes (Figure 5.12). The vertical deviation of the baseline unlike the undulations suggests that it is artefact. Figure 5.13 shows a baseline tachycardia with a rate of 150 bpm. There are no accelerations and careful attention reveals that the baseline

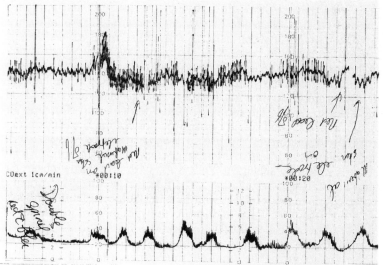

Figure 5.12   'Picket fence' artefact due to poor contact of a fetal electrode

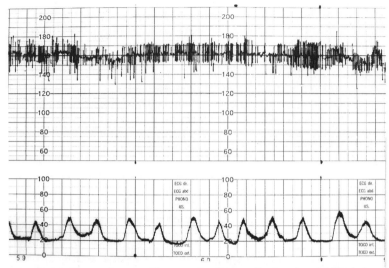

Figure 5.13   Abnormal trace with no accelerations and reduced variability being hidden by 'picket fence' artefact

variability is markedly reduced (less than 5 bpm) and is masked by artefact. This is usually thought to be due to poor contact of the electrode with fetal tissue or the absence of proper contact of the reference electrode (a metal piece at the base of the electrode) to maternal tissue. Although replacing the electrode and applying an adhesive skin electrode to the maternal thigh as a reference electrode may be of some help, usually these manoeuvres do not markedly improve the quality of the recording. In these situations it is better to record the FHR tracing with an external ultrasound transducer which has autocorrelation facilities. These fetal monitors give a good quality trace with a baseline variability which is equivalent to that which can be obtained with a scalp electrode. In the past when a good quality trace was not obtained with external ultrasound transducers the use of internal electrodes was advocated, whereas currently the use of external ultrasound transducers is indicated when the FHR trace with an internal electrode is not satisfactory (see Figure 5.11). Because of the good quality tracing obtained with fetal monitors using autocorrelation technology, there is no necessity to rupture the membranes in labour in order to place an electrode. The indications for artificial rupture of the membranes are during augmentation of slow labour and to inspect the colour of the amniotic fluid when a trace is abnormal. The 'picket fence' artefact can rarely be due to cardiac arrhyth-

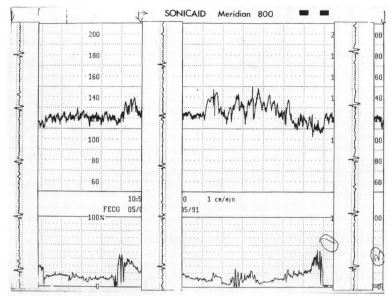

Figure 5.14   ECG signals on CTG

mias, and it may be useful to obtain the actual ECG signals from the fetal monitor. This can be obtained on the CTG chart paper with some machines (Figure 5.14), or it can be obtained by connecting a lead to a conventional ECG machine from an outlet in the back of the fetal monitor. If the 'picket fencing' has a regular pattern and the distance above and below the baseline is nearly equal throughout the trace then it may be due to cardiac arrhythmia. If not it is likely to be a problem with disturbance in the signal to noise ratio due to the electrode.

Other interference

Extraneous electrical influences can produce artefact in the baseline variability and if the disturbance exceeds the frequency of signals obtained from the FHR using a scalp electrode it can completely confuse the FHR signals with no FHR tracing. The use of transcutaneous electrical nerve stimulation (TENS) or the obstetric pulsar used for pain relief can produce this problem, and Figure 5.15 illustrates this with FHR tracing and the corresponding ECG signals.

With TENS external ultrasound monitoring is preferable.

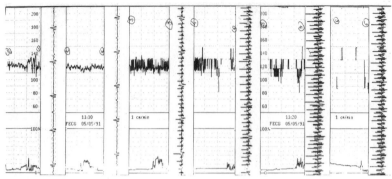

Figure 5.15   Effect of TENS on the trace as the TENS frequency rate is increased

Baseline heart rate: correct identification

Persistent accelerations may lead to confusion such that some traces have been termed 'pseudodistress' patterns. When the fetus is very active it may show so many accelerations that it is misinterpreted as tachycardia with decelerations (Figure 5.16). This situation can arise in the antenatal period or in labour. Certain clues aid correct interpretation. The clinical picture and risk assessment will indicate the probability of true compromise. Figures 5.17 and 5.18 show greater degrees of the same phenom-

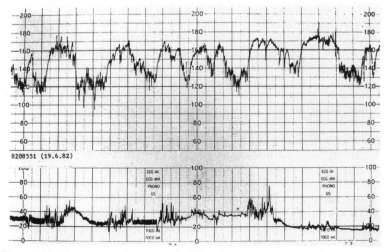

Figure 5.16   Very reactive trace: pseudodistress pattern

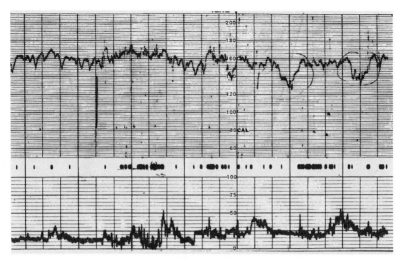

Figure 5.17   Continuous accelerations: very frequent use of event marker

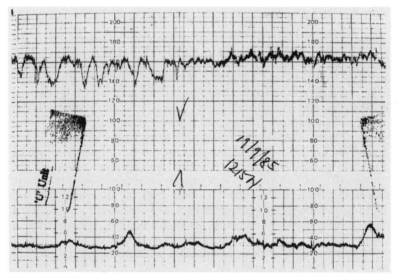

Figure 5.18   Confluent accelerations

enon and are more difficult to interpret. The trace may appear to show a long period of tachycardia and confluent accelerations. In the antenatal period, it is easier to recognize these patterns as non-pathological if the fetus is well grown, has a normal amniotic fluid volume and is moving actively during the recording of the

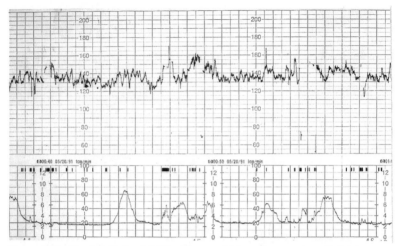

Figure 5.19   Hewlett Packard 1350 with a combi transducer; automatic fetal movement recording through the ultrasound channel

trace. This will be most obviously demonstrated by frequent use of the event marker by the mother or by evidence of fetal movements on the toco channel (see Figure 5.16). The Hewlett Packard 1350 monitor detects movements automatically (Figure 5.19). Such traces should have good baseline variability both at the true rate and at the higher rate. The true baseline rate on these traces is not below 110 bpm (the lower limit of normal for a healthy fetus). Inspection of the trace prior to the segment where there is doubt as to the true baseline rate would provide evidence of the true baseline rate. If such a segment is not available, continuation of the trace for a longer period should provide it. Repeatedly in clinical practice this pattern is misunderstood resulting in unnecessary intervention and the birth of a vigorous neonate behaving after delivery as it did before: Apgar scores of 9 and 10 after a caesarean section for 'fetal distress'.

A hypoxic fetus with a tachycardia with or without decelerations does not move actively.

At times there may be difficulty in resolving this issue. Figure 5.20a may be considered to show stress or a very active fetus. The tocography channel suggests rather frequent contractions, and after the reduction in the rate of oxytocin and contraction frequency a more understandable picture emerges (Figure 5.20b). Further evaluation may be necessary with biophysical assessment antenatally or fetal scalp blood sampling intrapartum. If an oxytocin infusion is in progress its rate should be reduced.

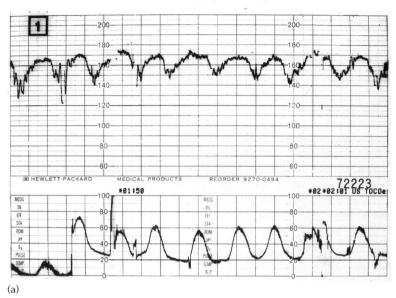

(a)

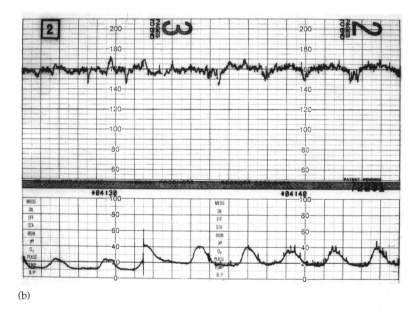

(b)

Figure 5.20   Trace showing: (a) hyperstimulation and tachycardia; (b) followed by reduction of oxytocin and resolution

Baseline heart rate: importance of recognition for each fetus

When a fetus is in good health the baseline FHR tends to vary by 10–15 bpm in an undulating way, slowing slightly in the sleep phase and after maternal sedation. It rises slightly during the active phase when the fetus moves exhibiting a number of accelerations. Gradually increasing hypoxia causes the FHR to rise gradually to a tachycardia. During the evolution of persistent repetitive decelerations, recognition of the steadily rising baseline rate due to compensation potentially leading to compromise is important. Each fetus has its own baseline rate and, although it may still be within the normal range for that individual fetus, it can represent a significant rise. It is important to take note of the baseline rate at the beginning of the trace and to compare it with the current rate. In the antenatal period comparison of the baseline heart rate of sequential traces has the same relevance. Priority should be given to the revised definition of normal baseline FHR, 110–150 bpm, bearing these considerations in mind. Any tracing with a baseline rate of greater than 150 bpm should be carefully scrutinized for other suspicious features. Traces within the normal range for baseline rate may be abnormal or ominous on account of other features (Figure 5.21).

A normal baseline rate can be associated with hypoxia and an ominous trace.

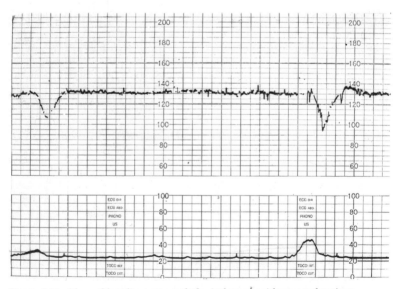

Figure 5.21   Normal baseline rate: pathological trace, with no accelerations, reduced baseline variability ('silent pattern') and shallow decelerations

Baseline tachycardia and bradycardia

A range of 150–170 bpm is termed a moderate baseline tachycardia and a range of 100–110 bpm is called moderate baseline bradycardia. Provided there is good baseline variability, accelerations and the absence of decelerations, these features do not generally represent hypoxia. Figure 5.22 shows a moderate baseline tachycardia but other features are reassuring.

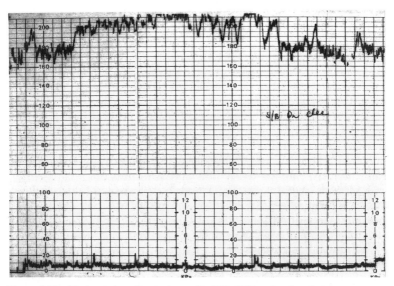

Figure 5.22   Moderate baseline tachycardia (150–170 bpm); other features are reassuring

Figure 5.23 is a rare trace showing sinus bradycardia at 80 bpm with a trace that is otherwise remarkably normal. The baby was born in good condition with a good outcome. The mother had had a renal transplant and was taking various medications including beta blockers for hypertension.

Tachycardia

Tachycardia with a baseline rate of greater than 150 bpm should prompt a search for other suspicious features such as absence of accelerations, poor baseline variability and decelerations. Tachycardia is not uncommon in preterm fetuses due to earlier maturation of

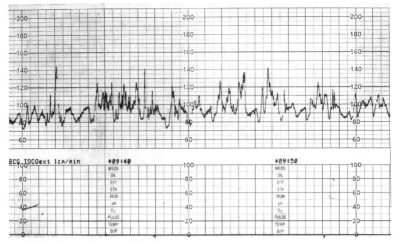

Figure 5.23   Sinus bradycardia

the sympathetic system. With increasing maturity of the fetus the baseline heart rate gradually falls and at term is often between 110 and 140 bpm. Fetal tachycardia may be due to fetal movement or increased sympathetic tone caused by arousal associated with noise, pain or acoustic stimulation. Fetal hypoxia, hypovolaemia and anaemia are pathological causes of tachycardia. Maternal sympathomimetic activation due to pain or anxiety may lead to fetal tachycardia as can dehydration leading to poor uterine perfusion. Pain relief, reassurance and hydration may be expected to reverse this. Administration of betamimetic drugs to inhibit preterm labour increases the sympathetic activity, whereas anticholinergic drugs such as atropine abolish parasympathetic activity through the vagal nerve resulting in tachycardia.

False or erroneous baseline FHR because of scale differences

In general electronic fetal monitors accept paper of about the same width; however, paper has been manufactured with different scales. In the UK machines have been calibrated to an expected paper display of 50–210 bpm with a 20 bpm per centimetre scale sensitivity. It is important this be uniform so that observers' perception of rate and variability is not compromised. Technically this could be solved by the manufacturers standardizing the aspect ratio irrespective of size of paper and paper speed.

False or erroneous baseline because of double counting of low baseline FHR

In normal circumstances the atrium and ventricle beat almost simultaneously followed by the next complete cardiac movement of the atrium and ventricle. The reflected ultrasound from these two chambers or even from one of the walls (atrium, ventricle or the valves) is used by the machine to compute the FHR. When the FHR is slow, at 70–80 bpm, there is a longer time interval between the atrial and the ventricular contraction. The machine recognizes each of the reflected sounds (one from the ventricle and the other from the atrium) as two separate beats and computes the rate, which may mimic the FHR as it will be in the expected range for a normal fetal heart. For most observers the sound generated will also give an impression that the FHR is within the normal range; this is because the heart sounds from the machine are always the same for every baby – they are electronic noise. During the false counting or 'doubling' of the FHR episode, listening with a fetal stethoscope will reveal the true situation. The suspicion that something is amiss will be aroused by the FHR tracing, which may show a steady baseline of 140 bpm but at times will be 70 bpm. Because it is a double counting phenomenon the upper rate on the recording paper will be exactly double that of the lower rate (Figure 5.24) and can be easily checked by auscultation. Such a trace can also be due to the machine recognizing an atrial rate of 140 bpm and a ventricular rate of 70 bpm at different times in a case with complete heart block. The mother may have an autoimmune disorder. Doubling the rate is a phenomenon dependent on the use of ultrasound monitoring. A fetal electrode will not show this effect and should therefore be used

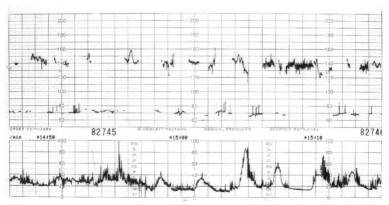

Figure 5.24   Intermittent double counting: heart block in maternal systemic lupus erythematosus

if in doubt. A situation of bradycardia with the doubling effect may be observed in a sick fetus as an acute episode and a preterminal event.
Beware of double counting.

Bradycardia: fetal or maternal

There is a facility, not well known and not commonly used, to record the maternal heart rate by using the external ECG mode of the monitor by applying skin electrodes, supplied with the equipment, to the maternal chest. The sounds heard and the trace obtained are identical to fetal recordings (Figure 5.25), particularly when maternal anxiety or betamimetic therapy for preterm labour results in a maternal tachycardia. If the woman reports with reduced fetal movements she may have a tachycardia due to anxiety, and this may be mistaken for the actual FHR while the fetus is dead. Note that the lower trace, which is maternal, accelerates and has variability as does the fetal trace (Figure 5.25).
Always use the fetal stethoscope before applying the machine.

When the fetus is dead the ultrasound may be inadvertently directed at maternal vessels. The technical quality of this trace is usually poor with incomplete continuity. In such circumstances it is prudent to verify the presence of the fetal heart activity by auscultation, confirming if there is doubt with an ultrasound scan.

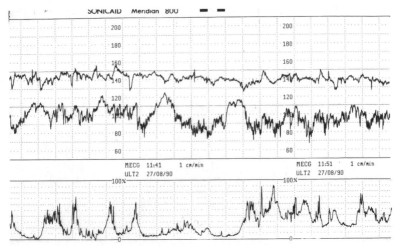

Figure 5.25   Fetal (upper) and maternal (lower) trace recording

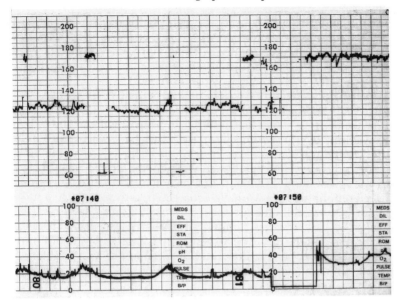

Figure 5.26   Maternal (120 bpm) and fetal (170 bpm) tachycardia ultrasound mode

If two baseline rates appear which do not show the 'doubling' phenomenon the transducer may be picking up the fetal heart at one time and the maternal pulse at another time. The trace in Figure 5.26 was recorded in preterm labour treated with betamimetic drugs showing fetal and maternal tachycardia. This should be verified by counting the maternal pulse at the wrist and by auscultating the fetal heart simultaneously. The findings should be documented on the CTG paper for clinical and medico-legal purposes.

Fetal arrhythmia

Complete fetal heart block may be recorded as a stable bradycardia and may give a trace as shown in Figure 5.24. Incomplete heart block is more of a dilemma. Both diagnoses should be substantiated by a detailed B mode ultrasound scan and further investigation. A heart block must be a proportion of the actual rate (2:1, 3:1) and this should be analysed. Confirmed heart block should prompt a search in the mother's blood for autoimmune antibodies even if she is asymptomatic. Fetal heart block compromises intrapartum surveillance and alternative methods to electronic fetal monitoring should be used (clinical sense, fetal blood sampling, Doppler blood flow study).

Occasional dropped beats or ectopic beats are a relatively common phenomenon in normal fetuses; however, more persistent arrhythmias can be associated with hypoxia.

Problems associated with interpretation of traces

In the past much time and effort has been spent on categorizing decelerations into 'early', 'late' and 'variable', rather than interpreting the trace as a whole in relation to the clinical situation. A given trace may be acceptable as normal in the late first stage but not in early first stage of labour. At times it is difficult to classify the decelerations as early, variable or late. Often they may have mixed features of variable and late decelerations. It is far more important to categorise any trace as *normal, suspicious* or *abnormal*. The FIGO recommendations have been given in Chapter 4, and for intrapartum use can be simplified and distilled as shown in Table 5.1.

Table 5.1   Classification of intrapartum trace

Normal
Baseline rate 110–150 bpm, baseline variability 10–25 bpm, two accelerations in 20 minutes and no decelerations

Suspicious
Absence of accelerations (first to become apparent, important) and any one of the following:

   abnormal baseline rate <110 or >150 bpm
   reduced baseline variability <10 and of greater significance if <5 bpm
   variable decelerations without ominous features

Abnormal
No accelerations + the combination of two abnormal features

   abnormal baseline rate and variability
   repetitive late decelerations
   variable decelerations with ominous features (duration >60 s, beat loss >60 beats, late recovery, late deceleration component, poor baseline variability in between and/or during decelerations)

Other specific traces categorized as abnormal are sinusoidal pattern, prolonged bradycardia <100 bpm and shallow decelerations in the presence of markedly reduced baseline variability (<5 bpm) in a non-reactive trace

---

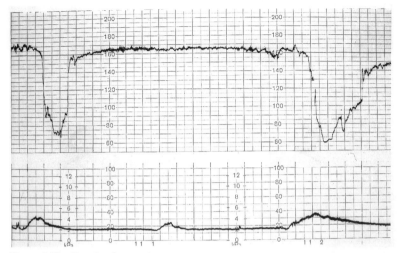

Figure 5.27   Grossly abnormal trace

Figure 5.27 shows a trace with tachycardia, no accelerations, reduced baseline variability and repetitive decelerations. Clinically the fetus is post-term and the mother is in early labour. This is a grossly abnormal trace demanding intervention. The decelerations may be analysed as variable because of the precipitous fall in the baseline rate characteristic of cord compression and because the decelerations vary in shape and size. They may be considered to be late because of the lateness in recovery. However, even when the decelerations are ignored the trace is abnormal because there are no accelerations, the baseline rate is greater than 150 bpm and the baseline variability is less than 5 bpm. There should be no hesitation in classifying this trace as abnormal. Those who have limited knowledge of the pathophysiology of fetal heart rate may spend time arguing about the nature of the decelerations without concentrating on the whole trace and the clinical picture. Intervention is mandatory.

Figure 5.28 shows an abnormal trace but is difficult to recognize unless one is aware of the exception to the rule of interpreting FHR traces. The rate can be within the normal range (110–150 bpm) but with reduced baseline variability (<5 bpm), and repeated late decelerations less than 15 bpm. This is an ominous picture unless the trace has shown recent reactive segments. The clinical picture has to be considered and at times an immediate delivery is opted for on clinical grounds. All the features of a given trace must be considered before it is categorized as normal,

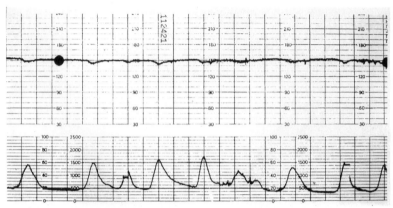

Figure 5.28   Grossly abnormal trace

suspicious or abnormal. The subsequent management of our patients depends on this.

- Accelerations and normal baseline variability are the hallmarks of fetal health.
- A hypoxic fetus can have a normal baseline rate, other features being abnormal.
- In the absence of accelerations, repeated shallow decelerations (below 15 bpm) are ominous when baseline variability is less than 5 bpm.

Chapter 6

Antepartum fetal surveillance

Antenatal care should be appropriate and effective. The low-risk mother will be seen largely by the midwife in community antenatal clinics. Higher-risk mothers will be seen in hospital antenatal clinics often by doctors. All require access to antenatal testing facilities. Recent years have seen a proliferation of maternofetal assessment units. The benefits of this include the gathering together of the various tests with the compilation and review of results. Daily outpatient assessment and review may be undertaken where previously admission to hospital was necessary. However, easy access may result in excessive testing with largely normal results. Protocols of referral should be formulated and audit undertaken. An assessment unit should be located near the ultrasound department because testing can be integrated with ultrasound examination. The focus of fetal assessment is the antenatal cardiotocograph (CTG). Appropriate equipment is the Sonicaid Team, Hewlett Packard 1351, Corometrics 118 or Huntleigh Baby Dopplex 3000. The Sonicaid System 8000 is an additional option which has a particular value in providing electronic storage of the CTG. Caution should be exercised in depending on computerized trace analysis with consequent risk of the loss of human skills of interpretation. A data collection computer has become essential. The unit should be staffed by motivated midwives who can diversify their clinical interest. They should have the support of available and interested medical staff in assessment of problem cases. The individual requesting the test should be aware of the result in order to plan and justify the further management. This should not be delegated by default to a junior member of staff.

Identification of the fetus at risk

There are two groups of women who may require fetal assessment:

1 Women with previously recognized historical risk factors such as previous stillbirth, neonatal death, or medical disorders such as diabetes mellitus, hypertension or other conditions.

2 Lower risk women who develop obstetric complications during
  pregnancy such as antepartum haemorrhage, hypertension,
  reduced fetal movement, intrauterine growth restriction or prolongation of pregnancy.

Adverse outcome due to prematurity or acute events like cord
occlusion or placental abruption cannot be predicted by existing
tests of fetal well-being. Fetal testing for the above indications can
only be for maternal reassurance and should be minimized;
excessive testing may generate anxiety. Chronic compromise due to
placental insufficiency operates through growth or nutritional
failure of varying degrees. Some of these adverse results might be
prevented by identification of the fetus at risk and appropriate
intervention. Hypoxia is not the only mechanism of compromise;
other conditions like diabetes mellitus, rhesus isoimmunization and
maternal or fetal infection may present a different threat. Selection
of tests appropriate to the condition is important. There should be
guidelines for testing which is related to the condition.
   Cases are referred for fetal assessment for a variety of reasons. The
most common indications are an abdominal size inappropriate for
gestational age and reduced fetal movements. Vaginal bleeding,
premature labour, prolongation of pregnancy and hypertension are
also common indications.

Fetal growth

The abdomen may be judged to be a different size from that
expected from the dates. More commonly this is smaller rather than
larger. The importance of detecting small babies *in utero* has been
emphasized in Chapter 2.
   The use of the term 'intrauterine growth retardation' has led to
much confusion with disagreement on how it should be defined.
The word 'restriction' should replace the word 'retardation' because
of the possibility of misunderstanding of the meaning of this word
by the woman.
   The clinical scenario may indicate a risk of hypoxic intrauterine
growth restriction (IUGR) in well-recognized situations: previous
IUGR baby, malnourished mother, smoking, alcohol, drug abuse,
medical conditions, gestational hypertension, multiple pregnancy
and other conditions. The measurement of the fundosymphysis
height (see Figures 2.1 and 2.2) in centimetres, given that the fetus is
a single fetus in a longitudinal lie, is plotted on a chart or simply
compared with the gestational age in weeks. If it is more than 2 cm
smaller than the gestational age before 36 weeks or 3 cm thereafter,
then it is *clinically small for dates* (SFD). The confounding effects of

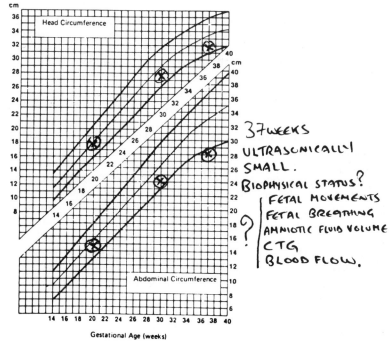

Figure 6.1 Ultrasound chart: small for dates

abnormal lie, obesity, fibroids, multiple pregnancy and poly-hydramnios have already been mentioned.

Clinically SFD is an indication for an ultrasound scan.

On ultrasound examination measurements of head circumference (HC), abdominal circumference (AC) and femur length (FL) are taken and plotted on a growth chart (Figure 6.1). The AC reflects fetal weight most accurately and if it falls below the 5th centile (Figure 6.1) this is *ultrasonically small for dates*. A fetus that is ultrasonically small may be an expected small baby – small parents and genetic smallness. However, an ultrasonically small fetus may be pathologically small due to an abnormal process. To distinguish one from the other the following should be taken into account:

- risk factors
- amniotic fluid volume
- subjective and objective fetal movements
- CTG
- other biophysical elements: fetal breathing, fetal tone, blood flow velocity waveform in fetal vessels by Doppler ultrasound.

Pathological smallness is what is generally referred to as intrauterine growth restriction. This term carries an implication of a likelihood of an asphyxial process being present. The pathology of growth restriction has more to do with function than with size.

Not all small fetuses are suffering from intrauterine growth restriction.

A growth restricted baby is one that has not realised its own intrinsic growth potential.

The growth restricted baby identified before or on admission in labour is flagged for special care with continuous electronic fetal monitoring, careful use of oxytocic therapy when needed and no undue prolongation of the labour process. The final proof of asphyxial intrauterine growth restriction comes from the neonatologist's observations of weight (in relation to expected weight for gestational age) and neonatal behaviour. Usually these babies have a scaphoid abdomen, little subcutaneous fat deposition in the limbs and can be recognized by measurement of ponderal indices.

Biophysical monitoring of fetal health

Fetal movements

Fetal activity in the form of fetal movement perceived by the mother is a reliable indicator of fetal health. Women should be encouraged to be aware of this. A reduction of fetal movement of concern to the mother is an indication for careful assessment, initially by CTG followed by an ultrasound assessment. An appropriate abdominal circumference and normal amniotic fluid volume on ultrasound are reassuring and often the fetus is seen to be active during the scan. The woman will also see this and be reassured. Commonly the fetus recommences normal movements and there is no need for further assessment.

In a randomized study involving 68 000 women, routine use of fetal movement charts was not beneficial compared with more selective use.[12] The commonly-used chart is the Cardiff 'Count to Ten' chart. Sadovsky, who studied fetal movement extensively, suggested that there should be four fetal movements in a 30-minute period during one day of which one has to be strong.[13] The expectation of four fetal movements in 30 minutes or 10 in 12 hours is arbitrary and correlated with good perinatal outcome.[14–16] A single fetal movement felt by the mother may not be recorded by the ultrasound movement detection devices. However, when a mother feels clusters of fetal movements for 15–20 seconds it is detected by the ultrasound transducer and is almost always associated with fetal heart rate accelerations (see Figure 5.19).[17] Women should be encouraged to be reassured by clusters of fetal movements.

The commonest answer to the question 'Is the baby moving?' is 'Yes, a lot'. We have to be prepared for the next question 'Can it move too much? Can this be bad?' There are many anecdotal reports by experienced clinicians of excessive fetal movements followed by death *in utero*. This must be due to an acute event and cord accidents or abruption could be postulated. *In utero* convulsions do occur whether due to pre-existing brain abnormality or another mechanism and may be reported by the mother as excessive fetal movement followed by death. In any event it must be excessively rare and this should not compromise our general reassurance of the mother that a lot of fetal movement is a healthy phenomenon. When a woman complains of excessive fetal movements a reversion to normal movements is reassuring but if there is subsequent absent fetal movements she should attend urgently for review.

Increased fetal activity can lead to confluence of accelerations mimicking a fetal tachycardia and the synchronous automatic recording of fetal movements as done by the newest monitors will help to clarify this situation.[18]

There are monitors using actograms that attempt to record fetal movement and fetal breathing in addition to the fetal heart rate. The clinical application of this principle remains to be proven.

Antepartum electronic fetal heart rate monitoring

Non-stress test (NST)

The recording of the fetal heart rate (FHR) for a period of 20–30 minutes without any induced stress to the fetus (like oxytocin infusion or nipple stimulation) to produce uterine contractions is called the non-stress test (NST). In the UK this is commonly referred to as an antenatal CTG. The duration of this test should be until reactivity is observed: until there are two accelerations in a 10-minute period. The sleep phase with no fetal movement and no fetal heart accelerations does not exceed 40 minutes in the vast majority of healthy fetuses and almost all healthy fetuses show a reactive trace within 90 minutes.[19] This forms the framework for extending the NST for 40 minutes when it is not reactive in the first 20 minutes. In some centres vibro-acoustic stimulus is used to provoke activity if there is no reactivity for 40 minutes.

A summary of the interpretation of the non-stress test based on the FIGO recommendations[7] and the actions that are recommended with each type of trace are given below.

Antepartum cardiotocograph (non-stress test, NST)

Normal/reassuring

- At least two accelerations (>15 beats for >15 seconds) in 10 minutes (reactive trace), baseline heart rate 110–150 bpm, baseline variability 5–25 bpm, absence of decelerations.
- Sporadic mild decelerations (amplitude <40 bpm, duration <30 seconds) are acceptable following an acceleration.
- When there is moderate tachycardia (150–170 bpm) or brady-cardia (100–110 bpm), a reactive trace without decelerations is reassuring of good health.

Interpretation/action

Repeat according to clinical situation and the degree of fetal risk.

Suspicious/equivocal

- Absence of accelerations for >40 minutes (non-reactive).
- Baseline heart rate 150–170 bpm or 110–100 bpm.
- Baseline variability >25 bpm in the absence of accelerations.
- Sporadic decelerations of any type unless severe as described below.

Interpretation/action

Continue for 90 minutes until trace becomes reactive or repeat CTG within 24 hours or vibro-acoustic stimulation (VAS)/amniotic fluid index (AFI)/biophysical profile (BPP)/Doppler ultrasound blood velocity waveform.

Pathological/abnormal

- Baseline heart rate <100 bpm or >170 bpm.
- Silent pattern <5 bpm for >40 minutes.
- Sinusoidal pattern (oscillation frequency <2–5 cycles/minute, amplitude of 2–10 bpm for >40 minutes with no acceleration and no area of normal baseline variability).
- Repeated late, prolonged (>1 minute) and severe variable (>40 bpm) decelerations.

Interpretation/action

Further evaluation (VAS, AFI, BPP, Doppler ultrasound blood velocity waveform). Deliver if clinically appropriate.

The antepartum cardiotocograph (NST) is usually applied for diagnostic purposes; its value for screening has not been proven.[7] Pooled results of four studies of NSTs involving 10 169 patients revealed a satisfactory outcome with a false negative rate of seven per 10 000 cases.[20–23] In order to reduce the number of non-reactive NSTs fetal vibro-acoustic stimulation to produce FHR accelerations has been employed.[24] The perinatal outcome based on the results of the FHR tracing obtained after vibro-acoustic stimulation has been shown to be as reliable as the results of the NST without VAS.[25]

The NST may be abnormal not only due to hypoxia but due to other causes associated with reduced baseline variability as discussed in Chapter 5. A review of the history with further evaluation will be helpful to clarify the cause.

Contraction stress test (CST)/oxytocin challenge test (OCT)

When the non-stress test is not reactive for 40 minutes or longer, it has been the practice in some centres to perform an OCT. It is carried out using intravenous oxytocin infusion starting with 2.5 mU/minute and increasing by 2.5 mU/minute every 20–30 minutes until three contractions are observed over 10 minutes. In cases of women with a previous uterine scar, oxytocin can be started at 1.0 mU/minute and increased by 1.0 mU/minute every 20–30 minutes. Absence of either decelerations or accelerations, or isolated decelerations make the test inconclusive. Repeated late or variable decelerations with at least half the induced uterine contractions indicate a fetus that may become compromised antenatally or in labour. Two accelerations in a 10-minute period and absence of decelerations despite contractions indicate a healthy fetus.

Comparative studies have shown fetal acoustic stimulation used to elicit accelerations in a non-reactive trace has a similar predictive value as a contraction stress test.[26] Compared to OCT, it is easier, cheaper, quicker and can be carried out in an outpatient clinic. It is also safer than OCT in patients with an overdistended uterus, with uterine scar and in the preterm period. Depending on the availability of other methods of testing of a biophysical nature, there is probably no place for OCT in current obstetric practice.

Assessment of amniotic fluid volume

Fetal urine contributes significantly to amniotic fluid volume. Fetuses with no kidneys have severe oligohydramnios. With diminished placental function and reduced renal perfusion the amniotic fluid volume decreases. Perinatal outcome is poor when the amniotic fluid volume is reduced at delivery.[27,28]

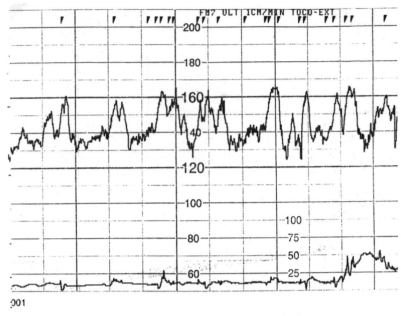

Figure 6.2   (a) NST in a postmature fetus: variability and fetal movements seen

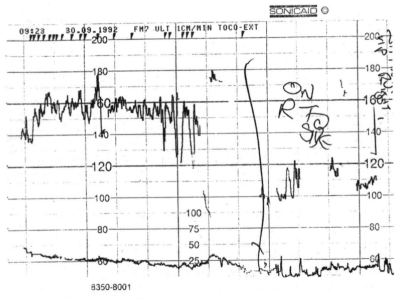

Figure 6.2   (b) Sudden decelerations

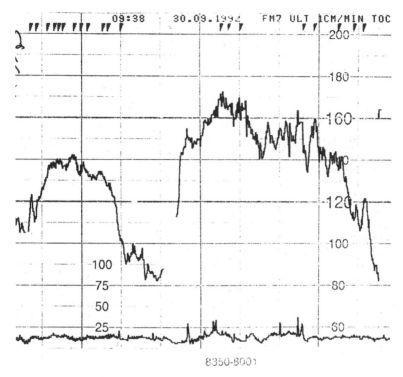

Figure 6.2   (c) Bradycardia and fetal death within minutes

Clinical evaluation by abdominal palpation can be deceptive. Impression of the amniotic fluid volume on ultrasound examination is fairly reliable. Objective assessment of the vertical depth of the largest pocket of amniotic fluid after excluding loops of cord or the sum of the vertical pockets in the four quadrants of the uterus (amniotic fluid index = AFI) is used in practice. The AFI correlates well with changes in amniotic fluid volume during the course of pregnancy[29,30] and there is little inter- or intra-observer variation.[31,32] The AFI is more sensitive in predicting fetal morbidity than the largest single vertical pocket of amniotic fluid.[33] An AFI of <5 cm is associated with poor fetal outcome[34] and delivery should be considered assuming reasonable gestational age. If only one vertical pocket is measured, a value of <3 cm in the largest pool is an indication for delivery.

In post-term pregnancy or that complicated by severe growth restriction, the decline in fluid volume can be up to one-third every week, and twice weekly assessment is advisable. Combining the AFI and NST with fetal acoustic stimulation (FAST) when necessary to provoke accelerations is one of the commonest first-line assessments in high risk pregnancies and is adequate for most women.[25] No unexpected fetal deaths occurred within 1 week of performing the test (AFI and NST with FAST) in a series of 6000 cases.[35] Antepartum fetal death within a week of reactive NST may occur for those who have an AFI below 5.[36] It is quite possible for a fetus with a reactive NST and good fetal movements to die suddenly in the presence of marked oligohydramnios (Figure 6.2). This may be due to umbilical cord compression. Most centres now recognize that for high risk pregnancies where a reduction of amniotic fluid volume is suspected (e.g. IUGR, post-term, etc.), it is desirable to perform an AFI. A schematic diagram incorporating AFI and NST with FAST as the first-line assessment is shown in Figure 6.3.

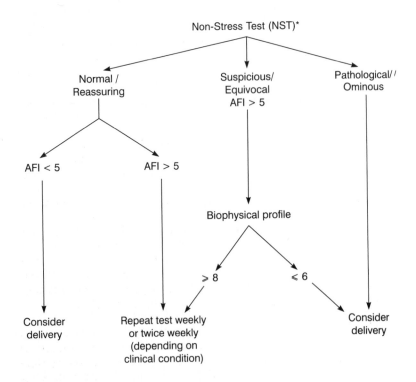

AFI – Amniotic fluid index
*Repeat NST and AFI weekly or more often according to clinical situation.
In preterm situations additional tests (e.g. Doppler velocimetry) may be of value

Figure 6.3   Suggestion for antepartum fetal monitoring in high risk pregnancies

Measurement of blood flow velocity waveforms

Sometimes it is not possible to deliver a fetus at risk of progressive hypoxia because of prematurity, although the biophysical profile, AFI and NST suggest possible compromise. Measurement of blood velocity waveforms in the umbilical artery and fetal aorta may give additional useful information for the timing of delivery in these circumstances.

Biophysical profile

The fetal responses to hypoxia do not occur at random but are initiated and regulated by complex, integrated reflexes of the fetal central nervous system. Stimuli that regulate the biophysical characteristics of fetal movement, breathing and tone arise from different sites in the brain. There is some evidence that the first physical activity to develop is fetal tone at 8 weeks' gestation. It is also the last to cease functioning when subjected to increasing hypoxia.[37] Fetal movements develop at 9 weeks and fetal breathing at 20 weeks. FHR activity matures last by about 28 weeks and is the first to be affected by hypoxia. In hypoxia FHR characteristics may become abnormal first followed by breathing, body and limb movements and finally by tone.

Evaluation of more than one biophysical parameter to assess fetal health has been suggested but it may not be necessary if the NST is reactive and AFI is normal. In the assessment of biophysical profile, fetal movements, tone, breathing and amniotic fluid volume assessed by the scan and NST are considered and for each a score of 2 or 0 is given, there being no intermediate score.[38] When the NST is not reactive, as more often in the preterm period, it might be useful to assess the fetal biophysical profile. A score of 8 or 10 indicates a fetus in good condition. Retesting should be performed at intervals depending on the level of risk. In situations where the compromise may develop faster as in prolonged pregnancy, intrauterine growth restriction and prelabour rupture of membranes, it is best performed twice weekly. If the score is 6, then the score should be re-evaluated 4–6 hours later and a decision made based on the new score. When the biophysical profile is equal or less than 2 on one occasion or equal or less than 4 on two occasions (6–8 hours apart), delivery of the fetus is indicated if the fetus is adequately mature and has a good chance of survival.[39] Further evaluation with fetal blood flow velocity waveform measurement may be considered if the fetus is so premature that deferring delivery even by a few days is considered beneficial. Good perinatal outcome has been reported with biophysical profile scoring in high risk pregnancy[39] and as a primary modality of testing in prolonged pregnancy.[40]

A modified biophysical profile where only the ultrasound parameters are evaluated (without NST) has been found to be equally reliable.[41] Due to the time and expertise needed to perform a biophysical profile, many centres perform an NST (if necessary with FAST when NST is not reactive) and an AFI.

Fetal actogram

Three of the five features of a biophysical profile, fetal heart rate pattern, movement and breathing, can be assessed by use of an actogram. An actogram is a recording that can be obtained by a modified fetal heart rate monitor which will record the fetal breathing and body movements in addition to the fetal heart rate and uterine contractions[42] (Figure 6.4). Such equipment is being evaluated. If it is found to be reliable, 'biophysical profile' testing

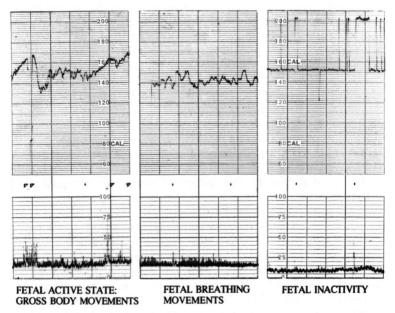

| FETAL ACTIVE STATE: | FETAL BREATHING | FETAL INACTIVITY |
| GROSS BODY MOVEMENTS | MOVEMENTS | |

Figure 6.4   Actogram exhibiting fetal heart rate and signals indicative of fetal body and breathing movements

would be easier, adding more information to the NST. With increasing hypoxia (as in IUGR) or when infection supervenes the fetus tends to reduce its fetal body and limb movements and its breathing movements. An actogram or biophysical profile done on a daily basis or every other day could suggest an increasing threat. The actocardiograph monitor is less expensive and the recording can be done with ease by a trained paramedical person, compared with the expensive technology and expertise needed to perform a biophysical profile. This approach might be attractive except for the absence of an amniotic fluid volume assessment.

Assessment of fetus in an outpatient clinic with limited facilities

With gradually increasing hypoxia, fetal heart rate changes take place first, followed by alteration in breathing movements, body movements and finally the tone. However, sudden demise can occur despite a normal FHR pattern when there is reduced amniotic fluid.[36] When there is fetal body movement for over 3 seconds it is associated with FHR accelerations.[43] The clinical outcome is similar when the NST is reactive with or without FAST to produce accelerations.[25] It is therefore possible to simplify fetal assessment at the outpatient clinic. A hand-held Doptone with a digital display will give a baseline FHR, and application of FAST at this time will result in maternal and observer perception of fetal movement and FHR acceleration, which will be displayed by the Doptone.[44] If the fetus continues to move, there will be further accelerations; in biophysical profile scoring, these two features (FHR accelerations and fetal movement) will indicate a score of 4. Since the tone is the last feature to disappear it is fair to give two points for tone when the fetal movements are plentiful with FHR accelerations observed on the Doptone. Low-cost printers are being developed which, when connected to a Doptone, can print an FHR trace similar to that obtained from a conventional CTG monitor (Figure 6.5). This enables the midwife to perform an NST in the home environment without difficulty.

Non-stress testing (NST) is usually used for diagnostic purposes and has not been proven to be of value as a screening test. The ability of the test to identify the problem being investigated should be known. A normal NST indicates fetal health/well-being. However, with chronic placental dysfunction, fetal adaptation occurs and normal (reactive) NST does not indicate the degree by which placental function may be reduced. Thus, the predictive value of a normal NST is governed by the clinical situation.

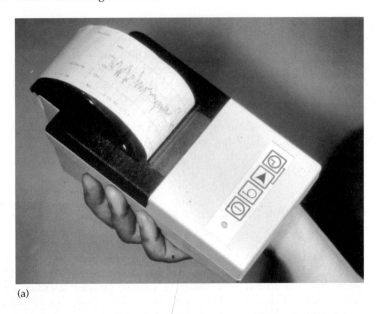

(a)

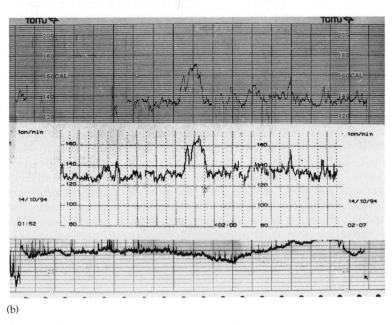

(b)

Figure 6.5 (a) Low-cost printer connected to Doptone; (b) an identical trace with a conventional fetal monitor

Case illustrations

The NST may not be normal due to a variety of causes other than hypoxia: cardiac arrhythmias, brain abnormality (congenital or acquired), chromosomal abnormality, anaesthesia, drug effects and infection.

Hypoxia

Severe IUGR is seen in the preterm period. It has been suggested that decelerations are a normal feature of the preterm CTG. There is a reduction in variability and lower amplitude accelerations are seen in the preterm CTG (Figure 6.6); however, major decelerations

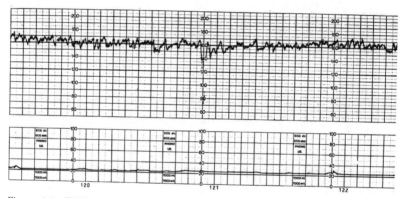

Figure 6.6   CTG in preterm baby: low amplitude accelerations and short sharp decelerations

are not a normal feature. In the preterm period short sharp decelerations mirror-image accelerations. They are often seen with change of sleep to wake state and may follow immediately after the acceleration. When major decelerations occur the clinical situation should be considered. Figure 6.7 is from a known case of severe intrauterine growth restriction at 25 weeks' gestation. There was oligohydramnios, poor fetal movement and very abnormal fetal and maternal blood flow. On account of a very small fetal weight estimate and early gestation the couple, with the advice of the obstetrician, opted for conservative management. The fetus died *in utero* 3 days later. Given a bigger weight estimate and later gestation, delivery would have been appropriate. There will be no guarantee that the baby is not already damaged; however, there is a

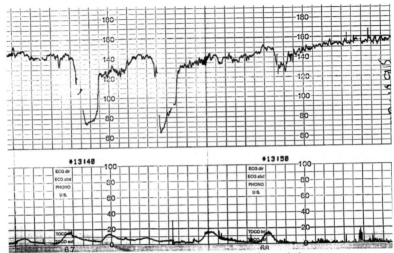

Figure 6.7   NST in a case of severe intrauterine growth restriction, oligohydramnios, poor fetal movement and abnormal fetal and abnormal maternal blood flow

good chance a bigger more mature baby will do well with good neonatal intensive care.[45] Leaving a fetus to die *in utero* is difficult in the face of reasonable weight and gestation.

Cardiac arrhythmias

Fetal arrhythmia may give rise to an abnormal trace, although the fetus is not hypoxic. Figure 6.8a was obtained from a case where the midwife auscultated the fetal heart in the antenatal clinic and heard a tachycardia. She noted that the multiparous woman was classically low risk and that the fetus was well grown and moving. This was confirmed by ultrasound scan after referral to hospital. Twenty hours later the CTG was repeated and was essentially unchanged. Advice was sought from a specialized unit, a diagnosis of fetal supraventricular tachycardia was made and the administration of double the adult dose of digoxin was recommended. Fetal echocardiography was normal. Figure 6.8b was recorded the following day. The pregnancy continued culminating in normal labour, normal intrapartum CTG, and normal delivery of a healthy baby 2 weeks later. The baby had a structurally normal heart and no further problem with the heart rhythm. Figure 6.9 is a similar case but the observation of supraventricular tachycardia was made in early labour. Advice was sought and the administration of digoxin

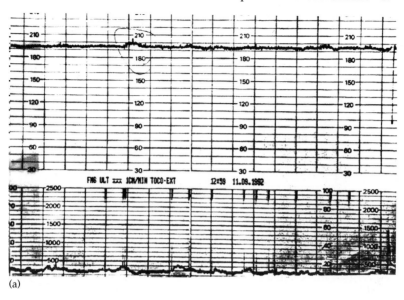

(a)

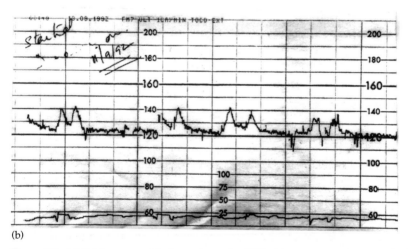

(b)

Figure 6.8 (a) Fetal supraventricular tachycardia (SVT); (b) reversal to normal rate after maternal administration of digoxin

considered inappropriate because the drug would not have taken effect until after the baby had been born. The baby was noted to be moving and continued to do so during labour. The amniotic fluid was clear and the woman was low risk. The CTG remained unchanged during the 6 hours of labour until the second stage. At

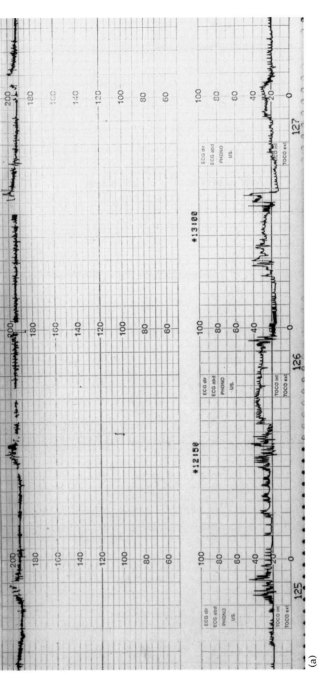

Figure 6.9 (a) SVT diagnosed in labour; (b) reversal to normal heart rate with decelerations in the second stage of labour

(a)

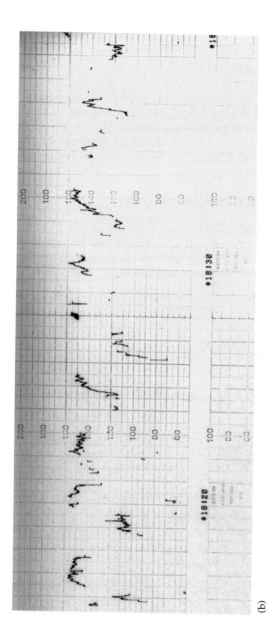

(b)

this time the features changed, possibly due to vagal stimulation with descent of the head. Although technically imperfect there appeared to be a normal rate, variability and second stage decelerations (Figure 6.9b). After delivery the baby had a normal heart rate and no further problem!

Heart block

This can be complete or partial, continuous or intermittent. Occasional dropped beats are frequent and of no significance: they generally do not interfere with the appearance of the trace or persist after delivery. A case of maternal systemic lupus erythematosus with fetal heart block has been shown in Figure 5.24.

Brain abnormalities: acquired

Physiological mechanisms controlling the fetal heart require the integrity of the central nervous system.

An abnormal CTG with no accelerations or decelerations and markedly reduced baseline variability was recorded (Figure 6.10a)

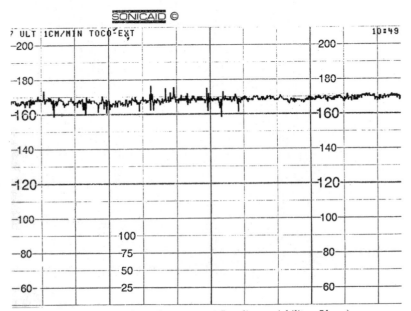

Figure 6.10   (a) CTG with a 'silent pattern' (baseline variability <5 bpm), no accelerations or decelerations

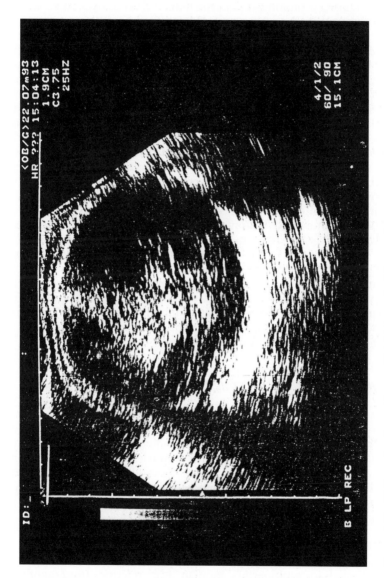

Figure 6.10 (b) Scan showing evidence of fetal intracerebral haemorrhage

when a high-risk woman on antihypertensive medication presented with a sudden cessation of fetal movement. The fetus was well grown and the amniotic fluid volume was normal on ultrasound scan. During a prolonged scan the fetus did not move. There was a collapsed stomach and an atonic dilated bladder with evidence of a large cerebral haemorrhage (Figure 6.10b). In view of the unusual findings a fetal blood sample was obtained from the umbilical vein for karyotyping, fetal haematology and cytomegalovirus screening. The fetal blood gases were normal and the fetal haemoglobin was 8 g/dl (1.24 mmol/l) consistent with the intracranial haemorrhage. While the karyotype results were awaited the fetus did not move and died 24 hours after the procedure. Post-mortem confirmed the cerebral haemorrhage. This severely 'brain-damaged' fetus was not hypoxic and if delivered would have had a very poor prognosis. The mother accepted and understood the outcome: she has since had a living child. Intracranial haemorrhage may occur in cases of alloimmune thrombocytopenia or when the woman is on warfarin therapy. When a CTG becomes abnormal despite good growth and good amniotic fluid volume such unusual causes must be considered before deciding to deliver. Delivery will not lead to an improved outcome in these circumstances. In twin-to-twin transfusion syndrome when one fetus dies, the 'second fetus' may suffer from the consequences of sudden haemodynamic changes which may affect the brain and then manifest as a non-reactive CTG. No changes in blood gases on fetal blood sampling or obvious ultrasonic morphological change in the brain are seen immediately but vacuolation in the brain may follow.

Brain abnormalities: congenital

The inability to maintain a steady baseline heart rate (Figure 6.11a) can be due to severe hypoxic brain damage or may be associated with severe brain malformation. If the fetus is active, indicated by fetal movements, it is unlikely to be hypoxic and the cause of such a trace should be sought by further investigation. The associated pathology was holoprosencephaly shown by ultrasound examination (Figure 6.11b).

Chromosomal abnormality

A 39-year-old multiparous woman was referred from another hospital with a well-grown fetus, reduced fetal movements, and a good volume of amniotic fluid and yet an abnormal CTG (Figure 6.12). The Doppler blood flow studies in fetus and mother were

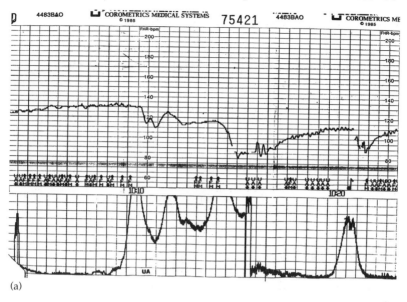

(a)

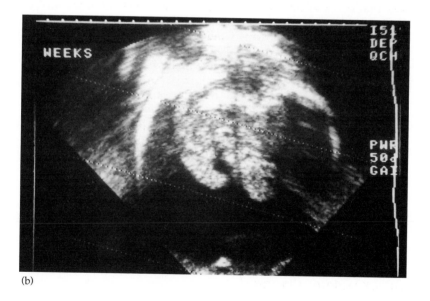

(b)

Figure 6.11   (a) CTG: unsteady baseline but with plenty of fetal movement; (b) Scan showing the fetus with holoprosencephaly

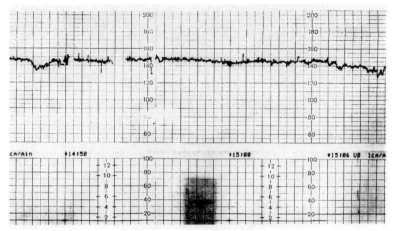

Figure 6.12   CTG with poor baseline variability, no accelerations and isolated decelerations. Misfit of fetal well-being tests; abnormal karyotype

normal. There was a slightly reduced femur length and slight hydronephrosis. Delivery was deferred until the result of karyotype from a fetal blood sample was known. The fetus died *in utero* the day before the result, showing Down's syndrome, became available. The mother had been counselled of this strong possibility and requested the baby not to be delivered without the karyotype result.

In chromosomally abnormal fetuses, especially trisomies, the central neural pathway may be disorganized resulting in an abnormal CTG,[46] although the fetal growth, amniotic fluid volume and fetal movements may be normal. In trisomy 13 and 18 the fetus might be growth restricted with an increased amniotic fluid volume. In a proportion of these cases the CTG shows a steady baseline but with poor baseline variability, reduced or absent accelerations and isolated decelerations. The disorganized neural development may manifest after birth as mental retardation.

A misfit of fetal function tests suggests the need for further investigations.

Fetal anaemia

This may show a sinusoidal or sinusoidal-like pattern and is discussed in Chapter 10.

Anaesthesia

The fetus is anaesthetized as well as the mother! The fetus may excrete the drugs more slowly than the mother. A multiparous woman fractured her tibia at 29 weeks of gestation. She was given a general anaesthetic in order to insert a pin and plate. A CTG performed on her return from the operating theatre 2 hours after induction of anaesthesia showed a dramatic reduction of baseline varibility and the absence of accelerations (Figure 6.13a). The inexperienced junior doctor suspected hypoxia and thought delivery might be necessary. Ultrasound scan confirmed a well-grown fetus and reasonable amniotic fluid volume. The consultant recommended a repeat CTG 2 hours later (Figure 6.13b) and another 24 hours after that (Figure 6.13c). The pregnancy progressed normally to term without further complication.

Drug effects

Sedatives, tranquillizers, antihypertensives and other drugs which act on the central nervous system tend to reduce the amplitude of the accelerations and suppress the baseline variability. In these situations other forms of surveillance become necessary. With antihypertensive therapy fetal activity may be unaffected.

Infections

A fetal tachycardia associated with a maternal infection is a cause for concern. The mechanism may be direct fetal infection or secondary response of the fetus due to transplacental passage of pyrogens or adrenergic metabolites. When fetal tachycardia occurs with maternal tachycardia due to maternal urinary tract infection it usually settles with antibiotic treatment. However, when fetal tachycardia persists for a considerable period of time then the fetus may not be able to tolerate it. Consideration of the clinical picture will suggest whether an actual fetal infection is likely. Preservation of baseline variability and reactivity suggests a resilient fetus.

If there is reduced variability with or without decelerations in the absence of accelerations the fetus itself is sick. A mother was admitted at 33 weeks' gestation with a systemic illness and tachycardia. On assumption of the diagnosis of urinary tract infection a cephalosporin was prescribed. The trace showed tachycardia with markedly reduced variability and shallow decelerations (Figure 6.14). The mother's condition did not improve nor did the fetal heart tracing. Rupture of the membranes with the

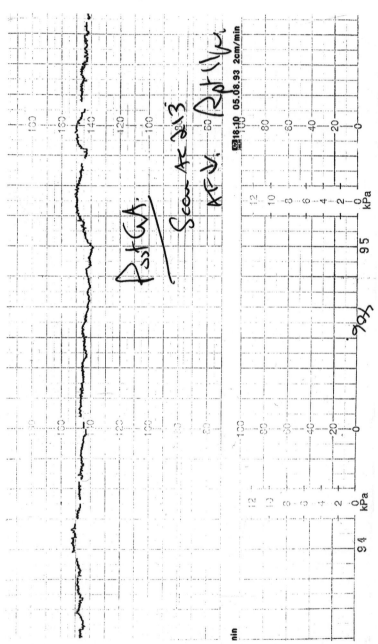

Figure 6.13 (a) CTG performed 2 hours after induction of anaesthesia: no accelerations and reduced baseline variability.

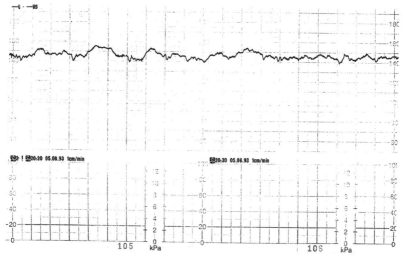

Figure 6.13   (b) CTG 4 hours after induction of anaesthesia

release of meconium-stained amniotic fluid prompted caesarean section. The baby succumbed within hours of birth to congenital listeriosis; it was heavily infected. This is reflected in the seriously abnormal fetal heart tracing.

Maternal illness and preterm meconium suggest possible listerial infection.

Suspicion of the diagnosis, blood cultures and treatment with ampicillin might have led to a better outcome.[47]

In cases with prelabour rupture of the membranes a CTG showing tachycardia, lack of accelerations and reduced variability suggests a higher probability of infection even in the absence of clinical signs.

Reduced fetal movements

This is a frequent reason for fetal assessment. A CTG on its own should not be taken as providing full reassurance in this situation. Even if the CTG is normal at the time of recording there might subsequently have been decelerations due to cord compression and oligohydramnios. Reassurance can only be obtained on this issue by finding a normal AFI of more than 8. A value of 5–8 is reduced and the test should be repeated depending on the clinical situation: generally in 3–4 days. If the fetal growth is satisfactory, AFI is normal and CTG is satisfactory no further assessment is

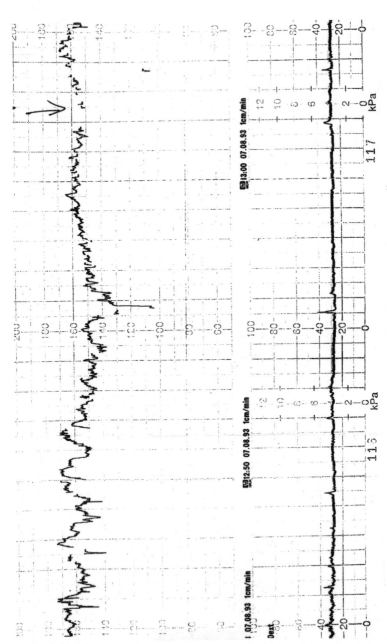

Figure 6.13   (c) CTG 24 hours later – reactive trace after the effect of anaesthesia has worn off

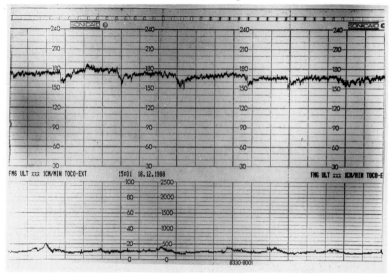

Figure 6.14 Ominous trace: listerial infection

immediately indicated. In such cases the movements frequently resume, often during the testing!

Prolonged pregnancy

This is a common indication for assessment in many hospitals. The clinician will have reviewed the menstrual and ultrasound dating and most cases will have reached 41½ weeks. The CTG may be normal but caution should be applied in being reassured by this. Figure 6.2 was obtained in the assessment unit in a case where the maturity was 42 weeks and 5 days. Two days previously the deepest pool of amniotic fluid had been 3.2 cm and the CTG was reactive. On the day of assessment the CTG was the first investigation to be performed. Fetal movements are seen on the trace and the first 7 minutes suggest reasonable baseline variability although a slightly fast rate. Deep decelerations followed and the woman was transferred to the labour ward. In the anaesthetic room 20 minutes after the end of the trace an ultrasound scan showed a terminal bradycardia. A decision was made not to deliver and the heart stopped within minutes of observation. The baby was found to be otherwise normal at post-mortem examination. Again the presentation suggests possible cord compression with oligohydramnios as the mechanism. In another case where intrauterine death occurred

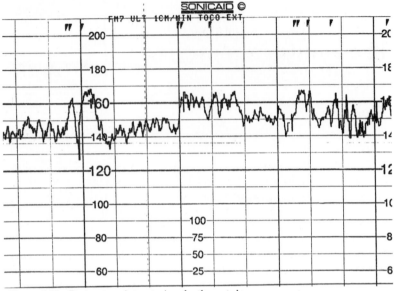

Figure 6.15   Postmature intrauterine death next day

24 hours after a CTG in a postmature gestation (Figure 6.15), the CTG had been normal and a single deepest pool of amniotic fluid had been 2 cm. Since that case we have performed AFI measurement during assessment.

The AFI should form an integral part of assessment of fetal well-being.

Chapter 7

The admission test

Fetal morbidity and mortality are greater in high-risk women with hypertension, diabetes, intrauterine growth restriction and other risk factors. A greater number of antenatal deaths are observed in this group. In term pregnancies morbidity and mortality due to events in labour are similar in those categorized as low risk compared with high risk based on traditional risk classification.[48-49] This may be because high-risk cases such as intrauterine growth restriction have been missed during antenatal care. With traditional assessment the fetal heart is auscultated after admission and every 15 minutes for a period of 1 minute after a contraction in the first stage of labour and after every contraction in the second stage of labour. During auscultation the baseline fetal heart rate can be measured but other features of the FHR such as baseline variability, accelerations and decelerations are difficult to quantify. Figure 5.28 shows an admission test of a fetus in serious trouble with an abnormal trace. Auscultation after a contraction by a skilled midwife (indicated by black dots) showed a 'normal' heart rate of 150 bpm.

Baseline variability is not audible to the unaided ear.

A new test is required to pick up the apparently low-risk woman whose fetus is compromised on admission or is likely to become compromised in labour. This is the *admission test*.

The admission test (AT) is a short, continuous electronic FHR recording made *immediately on admission*, and gives a better impression of the fetal condition than traditional assessment. In many hospitals electronic monitoring is performed but it is done long after admission. The mother may have waited for a bed, a nightdress, general observations to be noted and other administrative issues resolved. In most instances the mother walking into the labour ward is entirely healthy and her main concern is to have a healthy baby. An AT may identify those who are already at risk with an ominous pattern on admission even without any contractions (Figure 7.1). In those with a normal or suspicious FHR the functional stress of the uterine contractions in early labour may bring about the abnormal FHR changes (Figure 7.2). These changes

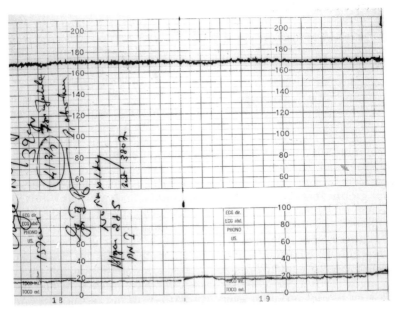

Figure 7.1   Abnormal admission test without contractions

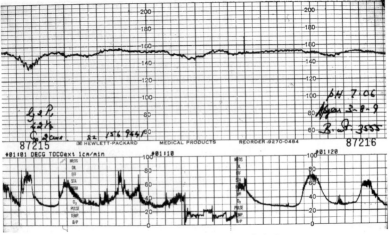

Figure 7.2   Contraction stress is often present in an admission test

may be subtle and difficult to identify by auscultation. Careful review may reveal a reduced FSH and a growth restricted fetus in such cases.

In Kandang Kerbau Hospital in Singapore an AT study was carried out on 1041 low-risk women.[50] An FHR tracing was obtained after covering the digital display of the FHR and the recording paper and turning down the volume so that the research midwife had no idea about the FHR trace. The transducer was adjusted based on the green signal light of a fetal monitor (Hewlett Packard - 8040 or 8041) which indicates good signal quality and produces a good tracing. The trace, obtained for 20 minutes immediately on admission, was sealed in an envelope and put aside for later analysis. These women were a low-risk population based on risk factors and hence were sent to the low-risk labour ward for care by intermittent auscultation. This study was accepted by the departmental ethical committee because our normal practice at that time was that none of the low-risk women had any electronic monitoring.

For this study a reactive normal FHR trace was defined as a recording with normal baseline rate and variability, two accelerations of 15 beats above the baseline for 15 seconds, and no decelerations. A 'suspicious' or 'equivocal' trace was one that had no accelerations in addition to one abnormal feature such as reduced baseline variability (<5 bpm), presence of decelerations, baseline tachycardia or bradycardia. A trace was called 'ominous' when more than one abnormal feature or repeated ominous variable or late deceleration were present. To evaluate the outcome, 'fetal distress' was considered to be present when ominous FHR changes led to caesarean section or forceps delivery, or if the newborn had an Apgar score <7 at 5 minutes after spontaneous delivery (Table 7.1).

In women with ominous ATs (n = 10), 40% developed fetal distress compared with 1.4% (13 out of 982) in those with a reactive AT. Of those 13 who developed fetal distress after a reactive AT, 10 did so more than 5 hours after the AT. Of the three who developed

Table 7.1   Results of AT in relation to the incidence of 'fetal distress'

	Admission test	Fetal distress
Reactive	n = 982 (94.3%)	13 (1.4%)
Equivocal	n = 49 (4.7%)	5 (10.0%)
Ominous	n = 10 (1.0%)	4 (40.0%)

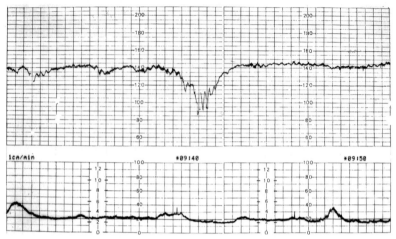

Figure 7.3   Concealed admission test of a fetus who died intrapartum

fetal distress in less than 5 hours, one had cord prolapse (baby born by caesarean section in good condition), and the other two fetuses were less than 35 weeks' gestation. They had low Apgar scores at birth 3 and 4 hours after the AT but needed minimal resuscitation. In those with an ominous AT there was one fresh stillbirth of a normally formed baby with normal birth weight for gestational age at term. The midwife was charting the FHR as 140/minute every 20 minutes for 2 hours when she reported that she was unable to hear the FHR. The admission test trace is shown in Figure 7.3. There is no doubt that the midwife's observations were correct; but unfortunately she could not hear the poor baseline variability and the shallow decelerations, which are ominous features, although the baseline rate was normal.

Barring acute events, the AT may be a good predictor of fetal condition at the time of admission and during the next few hours of labour in term fetuses labelled as low risk. Based on this, intermittent electronic monitoring for 20 minutes every 2–3 hours and monitoring by auscultation in between can be recommended in low-risk labour. If the AT is normal and reactive, a gradually developing hypoxia will be reflected by no accelerations and by a gradually rising baseline FHR; the latter could be picked up at the time of intermittent auscultation or electronic monitoring. Figure 7.4 shows sequences in an 8-hour labour showing gradual rise of FHR with absent acceleration and reduced baseline variability. Furthermore, it is known that if a well-grown fetus with clear amniotic fluid and a reactive trace starts to develop an abnormal FHR pattern

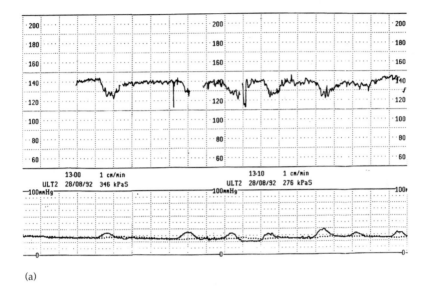

(a)

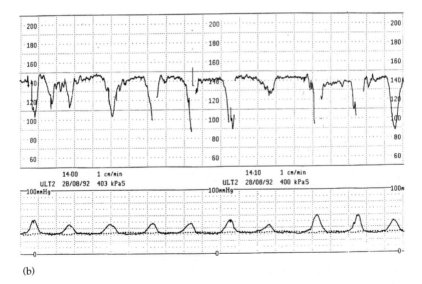

(b)

Figure 7.4   (a–f) Sequential CTG changes to abnormal

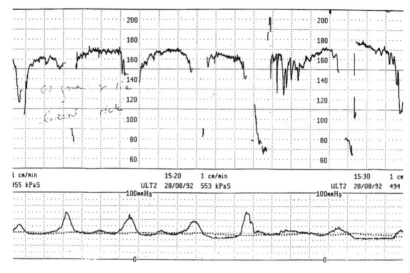

(c)

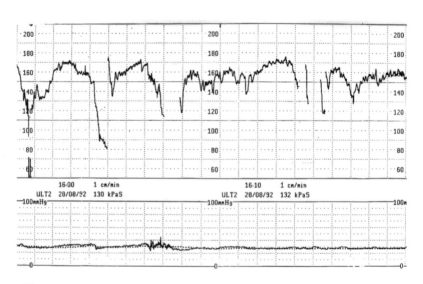

(d)

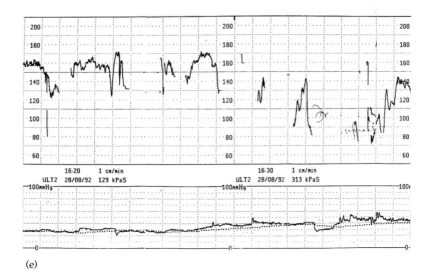

(e)

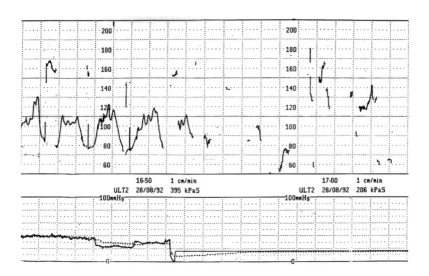

(f)

it takes some time with these FHR changes before acidosis develops. It was estimated that in these situations for 50% of the babies to become acidotic took 115 minutes with repeated late decelerations, 145 minutes with repeated variable decelerations and 185 minutes with a flat trace.[10] Therefore, it can be safely assumed that if the AT was reactive it is reasonable to perform intermittent auscultation every 15 minutes and 20 minutes of electronic monitoring 2–3 hourly in low-risk labour.

Other forms of admission test

The amniotic fluid index and Doppler indices of umbilical artery blood flow to assess fetal well-being in early labour have been evaluated as useful screening tests for fetal distress in labour.[51,52] These tests need expensive equipment and expertise compared with an admission CTG.

Assessment of amniotic fluid volume

Perinatal mortality and morbidity are increased in the presence of reduced amniotic fluid volume at delivery.[27,28] A reproducible semiquantitative measurement of amniotic fluid volume in early labour could conceivably be used as an adjunct to an admission CTG to triage a fetus to a high or low risk status in early labour.[53] In a study[54] involving 120 women in early labour it was found that ultrasound measurement of the vertical depth of two amniotic fluid pockets could be easily and rapidly performed by medical and midwifery staff and that the results were easily reproducible. They found that a vertical depth of two pools of amniotic fluid over 3 cm was highly sensitive and predictive when used as a predictor of significant fetal distress in the first stage of labour. In this study, six women had a vertical depth less than 3 cm; four of these women had a caesarean section in the first stage of labour for fetal distress and in three of the newborns the cord pH was <7.2. None of the women who had amniotic fluid volume greater than 3 cm required caesarean section for fetal distress. In a study of 1092 singleton pregnancies,[55] amniotic fluid volume was 'quantified' by measuring the amniotic fluid index (AFI), using the four quadrant technique.[29] An AFI less than 5 in early labour, even in the presence of a normal admission CTG, was associated with higher operative delivery rates for fetal distress, low Apgar scores, more infants needing assisted ventilation and a higher admission rate to the neonatal intensive care unit. When the admission CTG was suspicious, an AFI greater than 5 was associated with better obstetric outcome compared with those with an AFI less than 5. The low AFI of below 5 may indicate incipient hypoxia and the stress of cord compression, or a gradual decline of oxygenation with contractions in labour may be the cause of poor outcome.

Umbilical artery Doppler velocimetry

Umbilical artery Doppler velocimetry has been used as an admission test. It has been shown to be a poor predictor of fetal distress in labour in the low risk population.[51,56] A larger study of 1092 women has shown Doppler velocimetry on admission to be of little value in the presence of a normal admission CTG. However, in cases with a suspicious admission CTG, normal Doppler velocimetry was associated with less operative deliveries for fetal distress, better Apgar scores and less need for assisted ventilation or admission to the neonatal intensive care unit.[55]

Relationship of neurologically-impaired term infants to results of admission test

There is controversy regarding the value of continuous electronic fetal monitoring let alone an admission test. Other than acute or terminal patterns of prolonged bradycardia or prolonged decelerations of a large amplitude and duration there is little information regarding FHR patterns and neurological handicap at term[57-60] other than some observation of neurological impairment and non-reactivity,[61-63] especially in the presence of meconium. In a recent investigation of 48 neurologically-impaired singleton term infants, the admission FHR findings and the FHR patterns 30 minutes before delivery were analysed.[64] Findings of this investigation are shown in Tables 7.2 and 7.3.

Table 7.2   Admission FHR findings in 48 neurologically-impaired term infants separated on the basis of FHR reactivity

FHR pattern on admission up to 120 minutes	Reactive n = 15	Non-reactive n = 33
FHR variability (average)	14 (93%)	12* (36%)
Decelerations	2 (13%)	27 (82%)
Tachycardia	0 (0%)	6 (18%)

*$P < 0.001$

Table 7.3   FHR pattern in the last 30 minutes before delivery separated on the basis of admission FHR pattern

Admission FHR pattern last 30 minutes before delivery	Reactive n = 15	Non-reactive n = 33
FHR variability (average)	1 (7%)	11* (33%)
Decelerations	15 (100%)	5 (15%)
Tachycardia	14# (93%)	9** (27%)

*P < 0.05, **P < 0.001
#The baseline FHR in one case did not rise >160 bpm to be defined as tachycardia but showed an increase in baseline FHR of 25%.[64]

Based on the data in Tables 7.2 and 7.3 it is clear that all fetuses with a reactive AT (accelerations) will show the following features prior to or becoming hypoxic: all will exhibit decelerations (100%), almost all will have reduced baseline variability (93%), and tachycardia (93%). The one where the FHR did not exceed 160 bpm showed an increase in the baseline rate by 25% and decelerations which can be picked up on auscultation and action taken. On the other hand, if the AT is non-reactive the development of further abnormal features with progress of labour are variable and subtle; this is difficult to recognize by intermittent auscultation. This is because already there might have been hypoxic damage and the fetus is unable to respond. In those with a non-reactive AT nearly 82% had decelerations on the AT and 64% had reduced baseline variability (below 5 bpm) and many (82%) had a normal baseline rate. The fact that a hypoxic fetus can have a normal baseline rate and shallow decelerations of less than 15 bpm in a non-reactive trace when the baseline variability is below 5 bpm is not widely appreciated (see Figure 7.3).

All fetuses who exhibited a reactive AT had decelerations and a gradually increasing baseline FHR suggestive of developing fetal hypoxia. It is not difficult to identify this increase in baseline FHR on auscultation (Figure 11.13a–j). A recent randomized study compared the obstetric outcome in a group who had intermittent auscultation and 2 hourly 20 minutes of CTG following the admission test with a group who had continuous electronic fetal monitoring.[65] The obstetric outcome in terms of operative delivery, low Apgar scores and admission to the neonatal unit were the same in the two groups. The interval between admission to the labour ward to first detected fetal heart rate abnormality was the same in the two groups. This finding reassures that FHR can be confidently

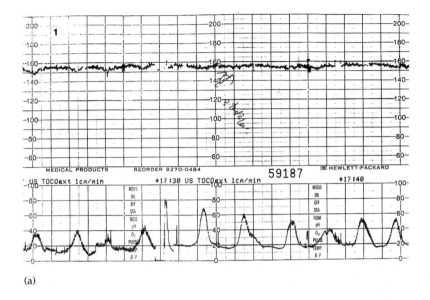

(a)

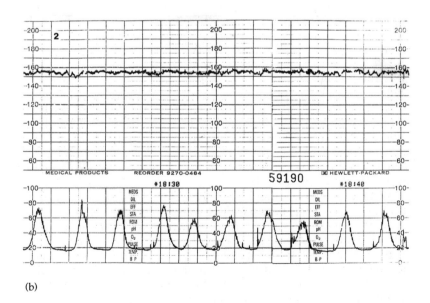

(b)

Figure 7.5   (a–j) Non-reactive trace with reduced baseline variability >90 minutes is abnormal even without decelerations in a non-reactive trace. Sequential traces until the baby's demise are shown

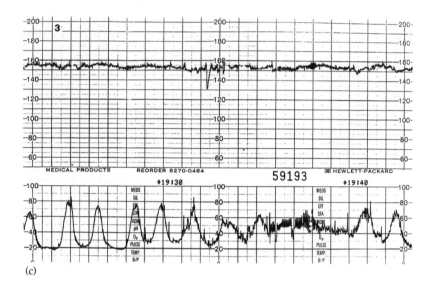

(c)

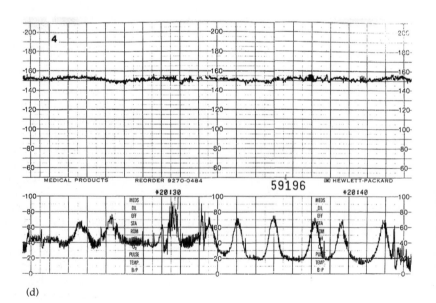

(d)

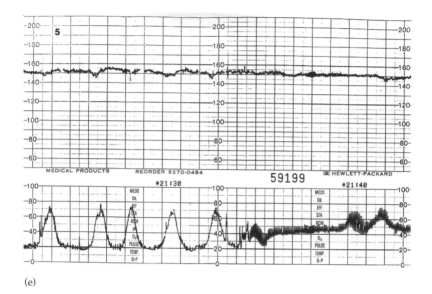

(e)

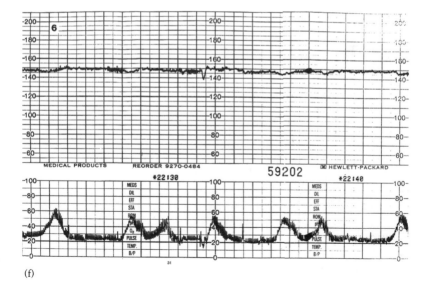

(f)

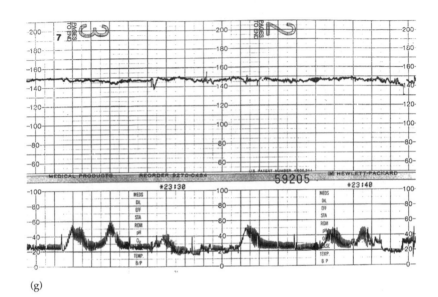

(g)

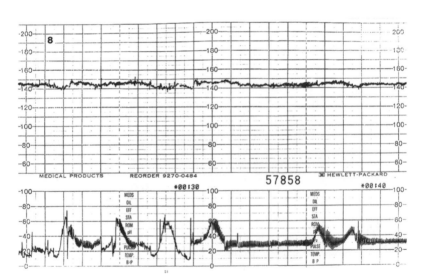

(h)

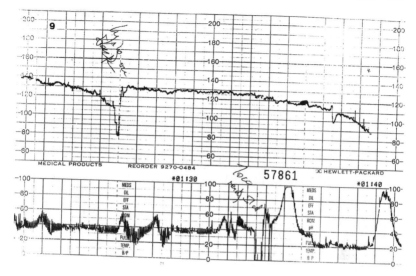

(i)

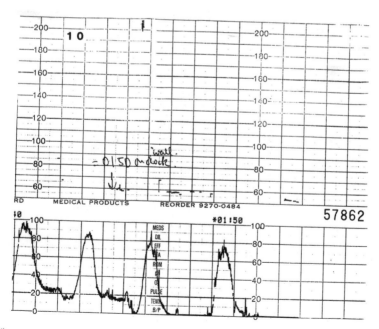

(j)

auscultated for changes that will indicate 'fetal distress' if the AT showed a reactive trace. On the other hand, if the trace was non-reactive with no decelerations and silent pattern (baseline variability below 5) for over 90 minutes the fetus may already be compromised or is likely to be compromised. Action should be taken to establish the acid–base status by fetal blood sampling or delivery should be considered. Failure to take action may end in fetal death (Figure 7.5a–j). It is difficult to know whether the fetus is already hypoxic or acidotic or is suffering from another insult (e.g. infection, brain injury due to haemorrhage, etc.) unless the acid–base status is known prior to or after delivery.

Fetuses with hypoxia may have a normal baseline rate, but with no accelerations, silent pattern (baseline variability below 5), and shallow decelerations (amplitude less than 15 beats) (see Figure 7.3). Such a fetus may not stand the stress of labour and may die within 1–2 hours of admission. Figure 7.6(a–d) shows the admission test trace with a baseline rate of 140 bpm. With progress of labour the baseline variability is further reduced (less than 5 beats) without a rise in the baseline rate and the fetus dies in a span of 40 minutes. There appears to be some difficulty in identifying the correct baseline rate and some may consider the baseline to be 120 with accelerations. Careful attention to reducing baseline variability would indicate that the correct baseline rate was 140 bpm with decelerations.

Planning management

An admission test is helpful when planning the subsequent management of the labour. High-risk women or women with suspicious or abnormal admission tests should have continuous EFM throughout labour. A normal admission test is an insurance policy that permits us to encourage mobilization with no further need to perform EFM for 3–4 hours or until signs of the late first stage of labour are apparent. Even in the second stage of labour a 1-minute strip of EFM after a contraction should be enough in the low-risk woman. Alternative delivery positions may be more confidently assumed.

A shortage of paper imposes a discipline requiring careful consideration. An admission test followed by monitoring in the late first stage and second stage, the time of greatest stress, appears appropriate.

How long should an AT last?

An admission test should last as long as necessary until it is normal. This implies a consideration of fetal sleep and fetal behavioural

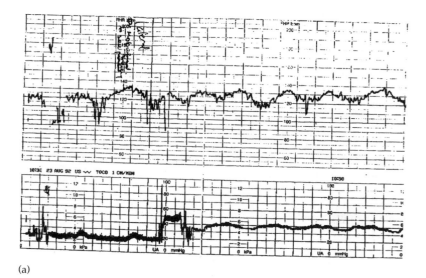

(a)

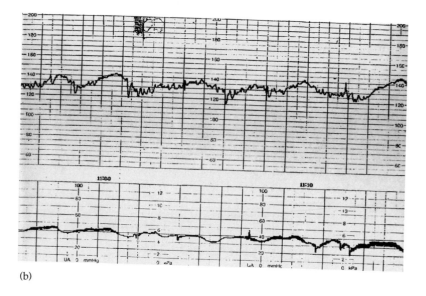

(b)

Figure 7.6   (a–d) A non-reactive trace with normal baseline FHR, silent pattern and shallow decelerations. Sudden fetal demise within 50 minutes of admission

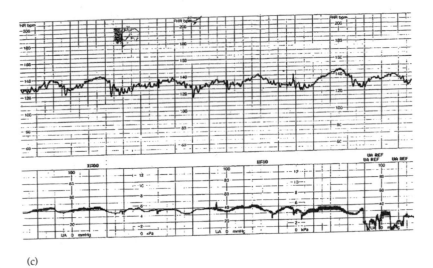

(c)

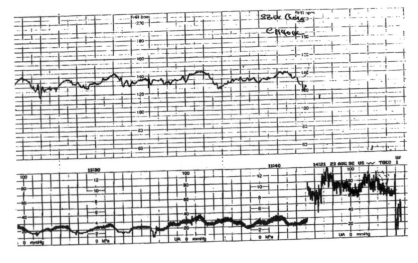

(d)

states. If two accelerations, normal rate and normal variability are seen in the first 5 minutes then that is very reassuring. It will be useful if two or more contractions are witnessed during this time as this will provide reassurance that there is no stress to the fetus with the contractions. If EFM is commenced at the start of a quiescent phase for the fetus then it will need to continue until the fetus reawakes. Most ATs should last 15–30 minutes; however, the mother with a normal trace in 5 minutes, keen for mobilization and natural labour should not be monitored unduly. Midwives can gain more confidence in the home birth situation by applying these principles and using a hand held Doptone and, if necessary, a connected printer.

EFM should be appropriate: not too much, not too little.

Chapter 8

Cardiotocographic interpretation: clinical scenarios

Meconium-stained amniotic fluid

The significance of meconium in amniotic fluid has been often debated. There are two principal reasons why meconium is passed by the fetus: maturity and fetal compromise.

The incidence of meconium staining of the amniotic fluid increases steadily from 36 weeks to 42 weeks of gestation when it is in excess of 20%. This reflects maturation of the central nervous system and gastrointestinal tract manifested by increasing intestinal motility.[66,67] The passage of meconium by a preterm fetus is rare and characteristically associated with the unusual but lethal listerial infection.[47] Fetal compromise usually of an acute or subacute nature also leads to the passage of meconium. Very acute stress such as placental abruption or umbilical cord prolapse paradoxically does not often lead to the passage of meconium. There are various degrees of meconium-staining, ranging from diluted old meconium which is brownish-yellow to thick, green 'pea soup' meconium. Typically, thick undiluted meconium is seen in a breech presentation for mechanical reasons. Under these circumstances it is interpreted differently from the same appearance in a cephalic presentation. In a cephalic presentation the meconium has to find its way from the fetal anus near the fundus of the uterus to the cervix and vagina; it has to pass through the uterine cavity which is normally filled by a good volume of amniotic fluid; this is the fluid for dilution. If there is little fluid then the meconium cannot become diluted and remains thick. If there is a good volume of fluid a greater degree of wetness occurs after membrane rupture, with thinner meconium. When membrane rupture occurs several days after meconium passage then the meconium is thin and old. If there is no amniotic fluid on rupture of the membranes then concern may be justified on suspicion of oligohydramnios. Thick, fresh meconium in a cephalic presentation suggests oligohydramnios and if the trace is abnormal then delivery should be expedited unless it is expected without delay. In The National Maternity Hospital, Dublin, on every bed side on the labour ward there is a specimen of that woman's

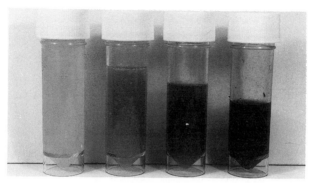

Figure 8.1 Meconium specimens

amniotic fluid in a universal container. This focuses the attention on the issues involved (Figure 8.1).

Clear amniotic fluid is reassuring.

Thick, fresh meconium in a situation of high risk is of great concern.

An attempt should be made in all cases with a fetal heart trace not classified as normal to release amniotic fluid from above the presenting part if necessary; this is done by pushing the presenting part gently upwards. If no fluid appears then the possibility of oligohydramnios and potential fetal compromise must also be considered.

Twin pregnancy

Perinatal mortality in multiple pregnancy is considerably higher than in singleton pregnancy, and particular risks are present during labour and delivery. Twins are generally smaller than singletons, with more pathological growth restriction. The second twin may be at greater risk of this and the ability to monitor electronically both twins continuously is therefore important. The latest generation of fetal monitors (Hewlett Packard 1350, Oxford Sonicaid Meridian and Corometrics 116) have been specially designed to perform this function. One twin can be monitored on direct electrode with the other on ultrasound or both can be monitored using external ultrasound. To have only one machine at a woman's bedside is a considerable advantage which should be fully exploited. The Sonicaid Meridian prints its own paper and therefore has the novel feature of a three channel trace (Figure 8.2). The Hewlett Packard and Corometrics models have a technique of printing out both

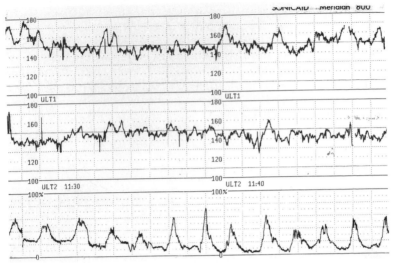

Figure 8.2 Monitoring twins – three channel trace (Oxford Sonicaid Meridian)

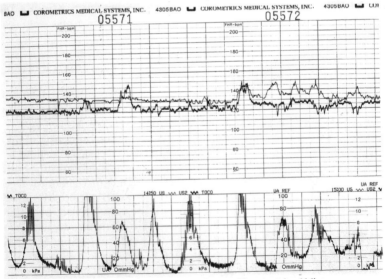

Figure 8.3 Monitoring twins – two channel trace (Corometrics 116)

traces in the same channel but in different shades (Figure 8.3). It is critical to follow the second twin with the ultrasound transducer: this may prove difficult especially in an obese mother. Assisted delivery is performed for the same indications as in a singleton pregnancy. A senior resident doctor must supervise the delivery of the second twin and ensure continuous electronic fetal monitoring during the interval between deliveries. Such an approach permits a more measured, less anxious delivery process; however, this should not be used as a justification for undue prolongation of the interval.

Breech presentation

Babies presenting by the breech are acknowledged to be exposed to more risks than those presenting by the head. There are several risks, but intrauterine growth restriction and umbilical cord compression have particular implications for fetal monitoring. The footling or flexed breech has a greater chance of compressing the umbilical cord. This is a classical scenario for variable decelerations due to cord compression as outlined in Chapter 4. There is also evidence that compression of the skull above the orbits by the uterine fundus is a mechanism for variable decelerations. Figure 8.4

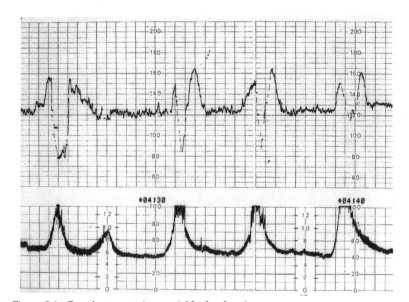

Figure 8.4   Breech presentation: variable decelerations

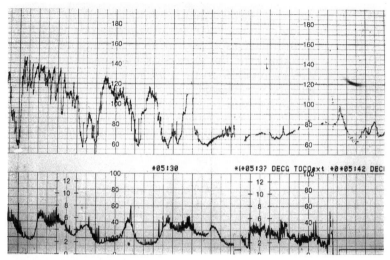

Figure 8.5   Breech cord prolapse

shows a typical pattern of cord compression in a breech. Should the misfortune of umbilical cord prolapse occur then the dramatic decelerative pattern shown in Figure 8.5 may be seen. The presence or absence of developing asphyxial features of changes in the baseline rate, baseline variability and magnitude of the decelerations related to the speed of the evolving labour process will relate to the outcome. Breech presentation presents special risks and in view of these there is little or no place for fetal blood sampling in a breech labour. The blood is more difficult to obtain from the tissues of the breech and it may be different from that obtained from scalp skin. If, having understood the normal mechanisms of CTG changes in a breech, there is a good indication for pH measurement then there is a good indication for caesarean section.

Brow presentation

Brow presentation in labour in late pregnancy is very unfavourable for vaginal delivery. The mentovertical diameter, which is usually about 13 cm, presents at the pelvic brim. This leads to head compression due to a mechanical misfit. Early and variable decelerations (Figure 8.6) are associated with this.

There are no typical features associated with a face presentation. The placement of a fetal electrode should be avoided in a recognized face presentation.

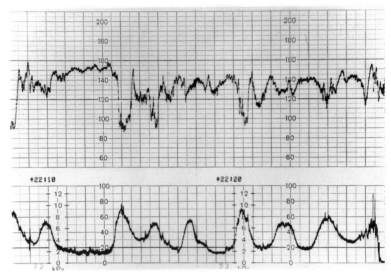

Figure 8.6   Brow presentation: decelerations

Previous caesarean section: trial of labour with scar

The stability of the placental circulation and uteroplacental perfusion is dependent on the integrity of the uterus and vasculature. With the dehiscence or rupture of the scar the major uterine blood vessels may become stretched and torn compromising the perfusion of the placenta (see Figure 11.4 a and b). There is also the possibility of the umbilical cord prolapsing through the dehisced scar giving rise to a dramatic cord compression pattern (see Figure 12.1 a–f). It is therefore believed that changes in the FHR as a result of this may be one of the first signs of scar dehiscence. The other signs of scar dehiscence such as scar pain, tenderness, vaginal bleeding or alterations in maternal haemodynamics are notoriously unreliable. Figure 8.7 shows a trace on a woman having a trial of labour with scar where, at laparotomy shortly after the trace, the scar was found to have ruptured. Figure 8.8 shows another trial of scar where emergency caesarean section was undertaken for prolonged bradycardia with a suspicion of scar dehiscence. The baby was delivered by immediate caesarean section (less than 15 minutes from the decision to delivery), had Apgar scores of 4 at 1 minute improving to 7 at 5 minutes, making a good recovery. There were no signs of placental abruption, scar dehiscence or any other explanation for the bad

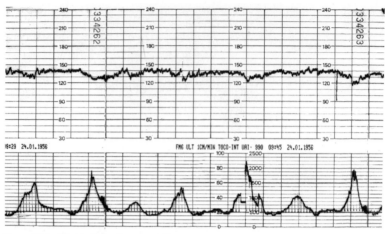

Figure 8.7   'Normal' trace: scar rupture

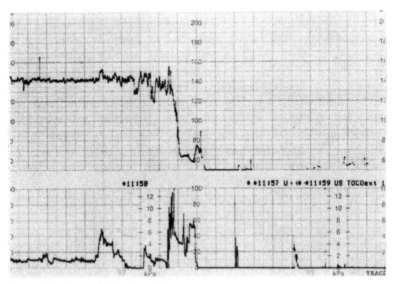

Figure 8.8   Prolonged bradycardia

tracing. Figure 8.9 illustrates another case where the fetus was already passing into the peritoneal cavity with a relatively normal trace and subsequently good outcome. Presumably there was some maintenance of placental perfusion. Continuous electronic FHR monitoring in a trial of labour with scar may be helpful in the diagnosis of scar dehiscence, although this is variable.

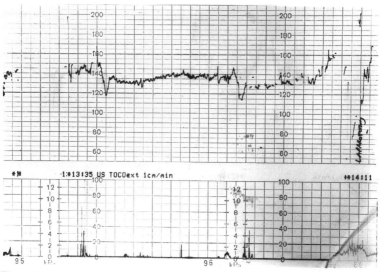

Figure 8.9   Scar rupture: relatively normal trace

Severe hypertension

Women suffering from severe hypertensive disease of pregnancy have at least two possible reasons for having an abnormal CTG. The first is the disease itself and its possible association with intrauterine growth restriction; the second is medication. Antihypertensive drugs by their very nature have effects on the maternal and fetal cardiovascular systems. Methyldopa leads to reduction in baseline variability and accelerations. Beta-blocking drugs result in reduced baseline variability and accelerations.[68] Figure 8.10 shows the trace of a fetus whose mother was being treated with labetalol for her hypertension; in spite of numerous fetal movements, accelerations are limited and baseline variability reduced. The picture is confounded by medication in these high-risk pregnancies, and complementary tests such as biophysical profile and Doppler studies are appropriate.

Eclampsia

A convulsion represents a major stress to the fetus which it may not survive. It is likely that such a fetus is already suffering from IUGR because of severe pre-eclampsia. Figure 8.11 shows a trace during an eclamptic fit. After any major acute stress it is important to check

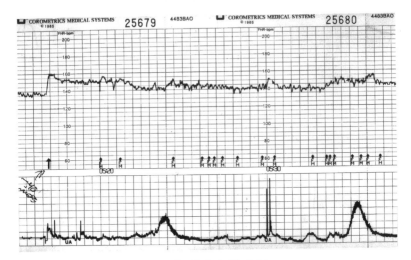

Figure 8.10   Hypertension treated with beta-blocker

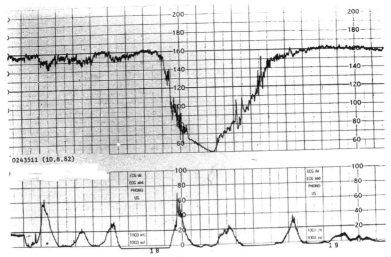

Figure 8.11   Deceleration: eclamptic fit

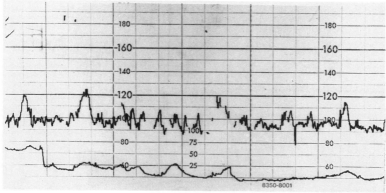

Figure 8.12   Unusual trace: multiple drug therapy

fetal condition by ultrasound scan or Doppler transducer of CTG before caesarean section.

Medication

High-risk women may be on multiple drug therapy. Figure 8.12 shows a trace from a woman with a functioning transplanted kidney who had been prescribed azathioprine, cyclosporin, prednisolone, antibiotics and atenolol. The low baseline is remarkable. Other tests of fetal well-being were normal. The trace remained normal in induced labour and the baby was in excellent condition at birth.

A baseline rate below 100 bpm in a non-hypoxic fetus is exceptional.

Epidural anaesthesia

The insertion of an anaesthetic agent into the epidural space can be associated with a degree of instability of the maternal vascular system. Providing the preceding trace has been normal then this represents a stress to the fetus that it can withstand. After attention is paid to the circulating volume and vascular stability returns then the trace returns to normal. This is a form of a stress test. However, it is wise to apply a scalp electrode before the manipulation for insertion of the epidural to facilitate monitoring if the preceding trace has not been normal. If the preceding trace has been abnormal then a more ominous situation may develop. Figure 8.13 is a trace erroneously not recognized to be abnormal before the insertion of the epidural. The cervix was already 3 cm dilated and the trace should have prompted membrane rupture which would have

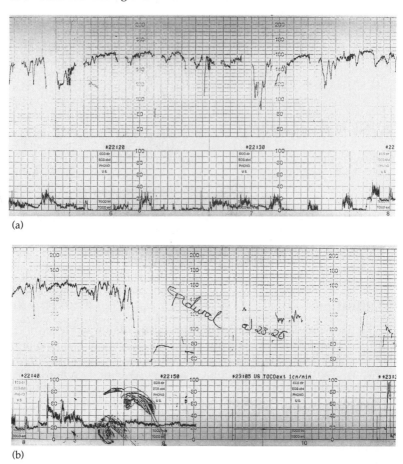

Figure 8.13   (a) Abnormal trace not recognized before insertion of epidural; (b) after epidural grossly abnormal FHR pattern, leading to operative delivery

revealed thick meconium and facilitated the application of a scalp electrode. Unfortunately, the stress of epidural insertion resulted in serious asphyxial CTG changes (Figure 8.13b) and the birth by immediate caesarean section of a compromised baby.

Second stage of labour

The second stage is a time of very specific changes in the mechanical effects resulting from descent of the fetus. In a cephalic presentation the initial appearances result from head compression. It is commonly seen in a multiparous mother in good labour that the onset of progressive early decelerations is a sign of the second stage before it has been confirmed by vaginal examination or the appearance of the head at the perineum.

Decelerations are common in the second stage.

Early decelerations gradually becoming deeper and developing variable features are characteristic of the second stage of labour. Reassurance is provided by a good recovery from each deceleration and a return to normal rate and normal variability, however short, before the next contraction (Figure 8.14). Under these circumstances assisted delivery is not necessary except for other reasons relating to maternal condition. Signs of hypoxia are gradual tachycardia, reduced baseline variability in between and during decelerations (Figure 8.15), additional late decelerations (Figure 8.16) and failure of FHR to return to the baseline rate after decelerations (Figures 8.17 and 8.18).[69]

Prolonged bradycardia necessitates delivery.

Failure of the FHR to return to the baseline and especially failure to recover to at least 100 bpm is a serious sign and delivery should be undertaken. Figure 8.18 is an example where the doctor was called within 3 minutes of a bradycardia. At that point the fetal heart then recovered. There was a further bradycardia of 3 minutes which did not then recover. At 6 minutes the mother was prepared, at 9 minutes the forceps were prepared and at 12 minutes the forceps delivery was performed with the baby born in good condition.

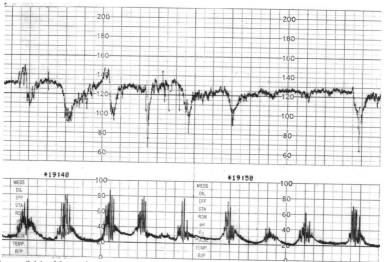

Figure 8.14   Normal second stage FHR trace: variable decelerations

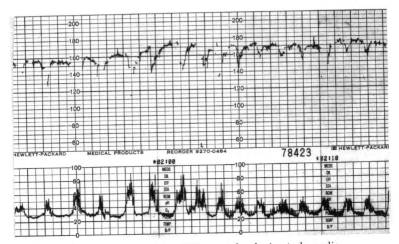

Figure 8.15   Abnormal second stage FHR trace: developing tachycardia

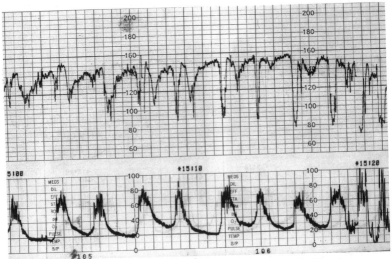

Figure 8.16   Abnormal second stage FHR trace: additional late decelerations

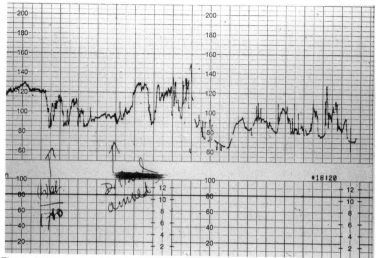

Figure 8.17   Abnormal second stage FHR trace: prolonged bradycardia

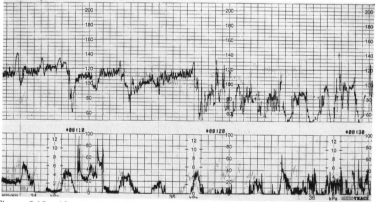

Figure 8.18   Abnormal second stage FHR trace: prolonged bradycardia

The 3, 6, 9 and 12 minute rule

3 minutes: call the doctor
6 minutes: prepare the mother
9 minutes: prepare the forceps
12 minutes: deliver the baby

A delay of 20 minutes or more may result in an asphyxiated baby.

Chapter 9

Contraction assessment

Effective contractions (the powers) of the uterus are an essential prerequisite for labour and vaginal delivery. The *progress* of labour, evidenced by dilatation of the uterine cervix and descent of the presenting part, is the final measure of contractions. During the journey through the birth canal (the *passages*), the passenger is intermittently squeezed and stressed by the contractions. Maternal blood flow into the uteroplacental space ceases when the intra-uterine pressure exceeds 30 mmHg. A well-grown fetus with good placental reserve tolerates this as normal stress and displays no change in the fetal heart rate. A compromised fetus may show changes with this stress. Oxytocin or prostaglandins are given expressly to increase the contractions; when they are given to induce labour the fetus is often already at risk. Particular care should be taken to 'manage' the contractions under these circumstances and to monitor the fetal heart continuously.

Recording

The commonest method of assessing contractions is with the hand placed on the abdominal wall over the anterior part of the uterine fundus. This permits observation of the duration and frequency of contractions. A subjective impression is gained of their strength. This is entirely adequate performed intermittently in normal low-risk labour.

Continuous monitoring of uterine contractions is performed using external tocography. The tocograph transducer (Figure 9.1) is a strain gauge device detecting forward movement and change in the abdominal wall contour on account of the contraction, recording continuously what the hand feels intermittently. The transducer is placed without the application of jelly on the anterior abdominal wall near the uterine fundus and secured with an elastic belt. It is important to adjust the tension of the belt for comfort and to secure an adequate recording. Obesity and a restless mother can compromise this. In these circumstances and in other clinical situations there may be a role for intrauterine pressure measurement using an intrauterine pressure catheter (Figure 9.2). This is the most effective

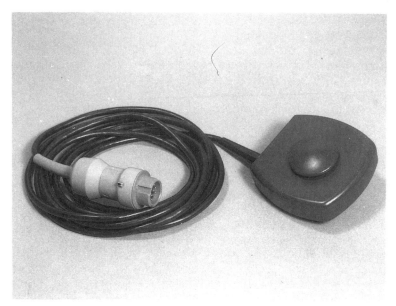

Figure 9.1   External tocography transducer (Hewlett Packard 8040)

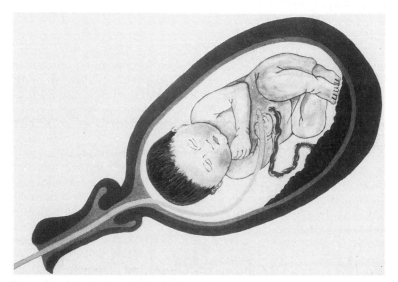

Figure 9.2   Intrauterine catheter *in situ*

method of recording contractions including a fairly precise measure of the strength in millimetres of mercury or kilopascals.[70] The technology for this has been developed in recent years with a disposable, solid state device now being available: the Intran II (Figure 9.3) (Utah Medical Products, Utah). Figure 9.4 shows the change in recording in an obese mother seen after converting from external to internal tocography over a period of 20 minutes.

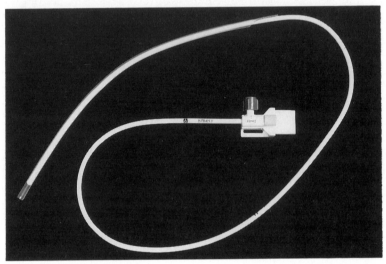

Figure 9.3   Intran II catheter

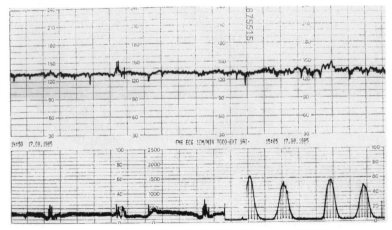

Figure 9.4   External tocography trace followed by internal recording

Measurement

What are normal contractions? The most relevant measure of contractions in labour is their outcome: dilatation of the cervix and descent of the presenting part. The quality of contractions present is very variable. A simple assessment of the frequency of contractions (number per 10 minutes), the mean duration (in seconds) and a subjective impression of strength (weak, moderate or strong) usually suffices. The method of recording this is seen on the partogram (see Figure 2.3). When intrauterine pressure monitoring is being used the opportunity arises for greater precision. In 1957 Caldeyro-Barcia suggested Montevideo units using average pressure multiplied by frequency.[71] In 1973 Hon and Paul introduced the concept of contraction area under the curve: uterine activity units.[72] In 1977 Steer introduced the active contractions area under the curve: kilopascal seconds per 15 minutes.[73] A simple system based on Système Internationale (SI) units has been considered and recommended by the Royal College of Obstetrics and Gynaecologists Working Party on Cardiotocograph Technology.[74]

The appropriate units for intrauterine pressure quantification are listed in Table 9.1, and the appropriate units for measuring the total activity over a period of time are listed in Table 9.2. The recommended period of measurement is 15 minutes.

Consistent terminology is essential.

Table 9.1   Units for intrauterine pressure quantification

Mean contraction active pressure (MCAP)	kPa
Mean baseline pressure	kPa
Mean contraction frequency	number per 10 minutes
Mean duration of contractions	seconds
Mean active pressure (MAP): sum of MCAP divided by time	kPa

Table 9.2   Units for measuring the total activity over a period of time

Active pressure integral (API)	kPas
Baseline pressure integral (BPI)	kPas
Number of contractions per period	
Total duration of contractions	seconds
Proportion of active time	per cent

Clinical application

What are the indications for continuous tocography? In general, continuous external tocography is performed when continuous fetal heart rate monitoring is being performed. This is a pragmatic, practical approach, although it ignores the rationale that the indication for each is separate although they may be related. If the FHR pattern is normal and the labour progress is normal then continuous tocography does not provide additional useful information, and the woman should be spared the discomfort of the tocography belt. There remains the issue that if the fetal heart pattern or labour progress becomes abnormal then information is already available about the pre-existing contractions: this is of limited importance. Nonetheless, established practice dictates that 2-channel monitoring – the heart rate and the contractions – is standard. Whenever the heart rate is abnormal or labour progress is abnormal requiring treatment, the need for contraction recording is clear.

Figure 9.5 shows an admission test performed on a woman with tightenings. Although the tocographic tracing suggests frequent regular contractions, the woman was not experiencing pain and did not go into labour that day. The tocography transducer may detect localized contractions that are not propagating throughout the uterus as also shown with marked irregularity in Figure 9.6.

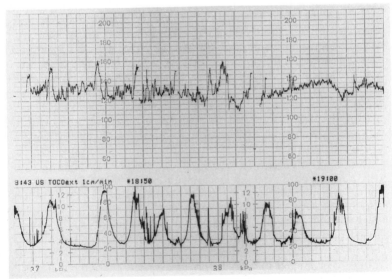

Figure 9.5   Contractions recorded: subject not in labour

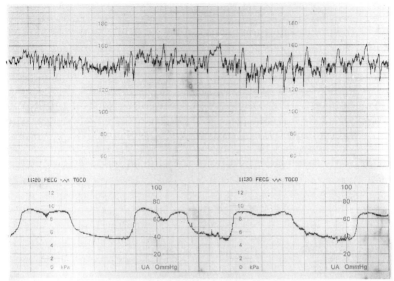

Figure 9.6   Contractions recorded: subject not in labour

The diagnosis of labour is not made from the CTG.
What are the indications for internal tocography using an intrauterine pressure catheter? Other than in an obese or restless mother, external tocography provides enough information to interpret an abnormal fetal heart tracing. The management of the contraction is another issue. If induction of labour or augmentation of slow labour (see Figure 2.3) is necessary then the more complete information derived from an intrauterine pressure catheter might be useful.[75] However, data now show that in most of these situations titration of the oxytocin infusion rate based on frequency and duration of contractions recorded by external tocography is adequate.[76,77] The exception might be the obese, restless mother or the nullipara with an occipitoposterior position requiring a high-dose infusion of oxytocin.

Breech presentation and labour with a previous caesarean section scar present specific problems. Some obstetricians do not practice vaginal delivery of a baby presenting by the breech; in those that do there is some reluctance to use oxytocin if labour progress is slow. The anxiety is that the slow progress is a manifestation of fetopelvic disproportion and therefore the sign to terminate the labour by performing a caesarean section. The counter-view is that poor contractions are just as likely (if not more likely) to occur in a breech presentation. If complete assessment of the fetopelvic relationship has shown favourable features and the contractions are shown to be weak then oxytocin augmentation may be safely undertaken. The additional information derived from an intrauterine pressure catheter may be useful under these circumstances.

A similar rationale applies to poor labour progress in a woman with a previous caesarean section scar. Additionally there is the further concern for the integrity of the uterine scar. Scar rupture or dehiscence may not manifest scar pain, tenderness, vaginal bleeding or alteration in maternal pulse and blood pressure; FHR or uterine activity changes may be an earlier sign of scar disruption.[78,79] Figure 9.7 shows a case where resiting of the catheter led to an acceptable

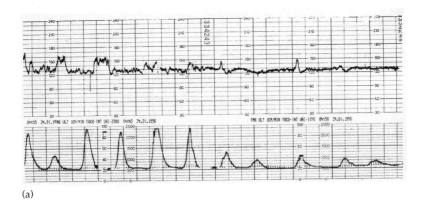

(a)

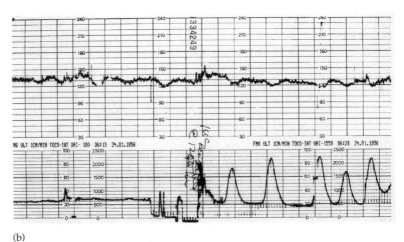

(b)

Figure 9.7   (a) Scar dehiscence: reduction in uterine activity; (b) intrauterine pressure catheter replaced in another pocket showing normal uterine activity

tocographic tracing in spite of scar dehiscence; presumably the replaced catheter was in a loculated pocket of normal pressure. In some centres there is a link between the indication for internal FHR monitoring with an electrode and internal pressure monitoring with a pressure catheter. There is no logic in this as each addresses separate issues. Excessive use of internal monitoring is invasive psychologically as well as physically.

There is a very limited place for intrauterine pressure measurement.

Uterine hyperstimulation and fetal hypoxia is a real possibility when oxytocics are used, and in these circumstances continuous electronic FHR monitoring is important.

The development of clinical skills and an educational motive remain important reasons for giving due attention to the contractions. In the USA many cases of litigation relate to the misuse of oxytocin. Better understanding of the labour process and contractions should help to counter such misuse.[80]

Chapter 10

Oxytocin and fetal heart rate changes

Oxytocin is commonly used for induction and augmentation of labour. It does not have a direct influence on the fetal heart rate or on the controlling cardiac centres in the brain as is the case with some anaesthetic and antihypertensive drugs. Its influence is indirect via increased uterine activity, mostly due to increased frequency of contractions or baseline pressure (hypertonus). Increase in duration or amplitude of contractions can also lead to FHR changes.

Figure 10.1 shows fetal bradycardia due to 'tetanic' or sustained contractions lasting for 3–4 minutes, caused by oxytocin hyperstimulation. Because the subject was a healthy fetus with a normal reactive FHR prior to the episode, the transient bradycardia returned to normal once the oxytocin infusion was reduced and the abnormal contractions ceased.

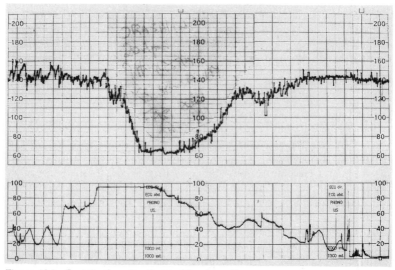

Figure 10.1   Sustained contraction and bradycardia

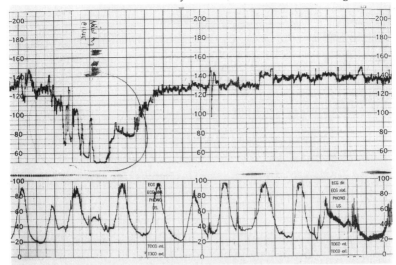

Figure 10.2 Hypertonic contraction and bradycardia

Figure 10.2 shows fetal bradycardia due to 'hypertonic' uterine activity. The baseline pressure was elevated by 15 mmHg for 3 minutes despite regular contractions. The raised baseline pressure reduced the perfusion in the retroplacental area leading to FHR changes which returned to normal once the baseline pressure settled to normal levels, restoring normal perfusion.

Figure 10.3 shows a reactive trace with one contraction in 3 minutes. An oxytocin infusion was commenced 10 minutes from the start of this segment at a rate of 1 mU per minute. This resulted in the late decelerations and changes seen in the latter part of the trace. The contraction recording shows no increase in frequency or duration of contractions nor increase in baseline pressure, but shows an increase in amplitude of contractions. Discontinuation of the infusion resulted in return of the FHR trace to normal.

The FHR changes associated with oxytocin infusion may be caused by the compression of the cord with contractions or by the reduction in placental perfusion due to increased intrauterine basal pressure and frequent contractions cutting off the blood supply to the placenta. Pressure on the head or supraorbital region of the fetus can also give rise to variable decelerations. The rate of increasing hypoxia would be shown by a deteriorating trend of the FHR. The rate of decline of pH depends on the FHR pattern observed and the physiological reserve of the fetus.[81] A rapid decline would be anticipated in post-term and growth-restricted fetuses and those with reduced amniotic fluid with thick meconium. Fortunately, in

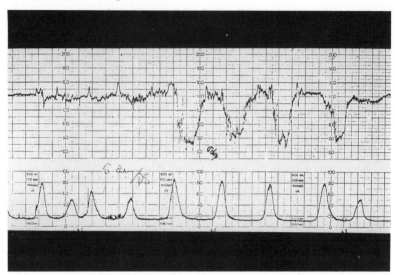

Figure 10.3   Normal trace and subsequent decelerations with oxytocin

the vast majority of patients who are given oxytocin, FHR changes of a worrying nature are not encountered and most changes, even when they occur, are transient and resolve spontaneously, or with reduction of the dose or transient cessation of the infusion. It is good practice to run a strip of CTG prior to commencing oxytocin to make sure of good fetal health as reflected by a normal reactive FHR pattern; if the trace is abnormal then oxytocin should not be used, as it can cause further hypoxia to the fetus by reducing the perfusion to the placenta by additional contractions.

If an abnormal FHR pattern is observed in a woman on an oxytocin infusion, the infusion should be stopped or its rate reduced, and the woman nursed on her side to improve the maternal venous return and thus her cardiac output in order to increase the uteroplacental perfusion. Oxygen inhalation by the mother and an intravenous bolus of tocolytic drugs to abolish uterine contractions are given in some centres. Such practice may not be necessary in the majority of cases and its value in the other cases is debatable. It is known that oxytocin becomes bound to receptors, and for its action to be reduced to half can take up to 45 minutes after stopping the oxytocin infusion. A case may be made for the use of a bolus dose of a tocolytic drug in a patient with a grossly abnormal FHR pattern.[82,83] There is little merit in performing a fetal scalp blood pH measurement in a patient receiving oxytocin since the FHR changes are iatrogenic. If the test is done soon after a prolonged bradycardia or after ominous decelerations, it may show acidosis prompting the performance of an emergency caesarean section (Figure 10.4a); on the other hand, if a fetal blood sample is not taken and time is allowed, the FHR recovers and within 30–40 minutes the scalp blood pH is likely to be normal (Figure 10.4b). On many occasions there is no need to measure scalp blood pH and the oxytocin infusion can be restarted after the return of the FHR to normal.

It is debatable for how long the oxytocin infusion should be stopped once the FHR abnormality is detected. It is usual to wait

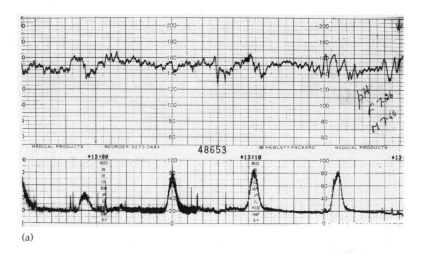

(a)

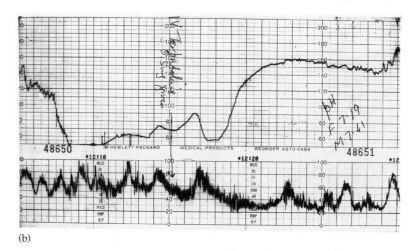

(b)

Figure 10.4   (a) CTG: bradycardia with acidosis and (b) reversion to normal pH

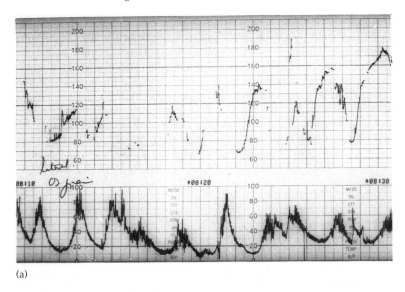

(a)

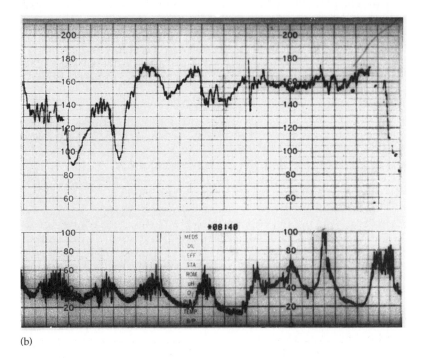

(b)

Figure 10.5   (a) Hyperstimulation and abnormal trace followed by (b) correction of trace after cessation of oxytocin

until the abnormal features disappear and the reactive trace is seen; however, it is known that although the trace is then normal, the fetal blood biochemistry reflected in scalp blood may still show a low pH, high P_{CO_2} and low P_{O_2}. Additional time is required for the blood biochemistry to become normal, which takes place rapidly once the FHR is normal. Noting the time necessary for the FHR to become normal after the oxytocin infusion is stopped and allowing an equal length of time to elapse before restarting the infusion would allow the biochemistry to become normal. Doubling the time period in this way before restarting oxytocin should cause no or little FHR changes compared with restarting oxytocin immediately the FHR returns to normal. It is also advisable to resume the infusion at half the previous dose rate to reduce the chances of hyperstimulation or abnormal FHR changes. Since the sensitivity of the uterus to oxytocin increases with progress of labour,[84] such careful titration is likely to produce fewer problems of abnormal FHR changes or uterine hyperstimulation.

Figure 10.5a shows abnormal FHR changes produced by oxytocic hyperstimulation. Even with immediate cessation of oxytocin infusion it takes about 45 minutes for the FHR to return to normal (Figure 10.5b) and hence sufficient time should be given for recovery. Although it is advisable to stop the oxytocin infusion as soon as abnormal FHR patterns such as decelerations or bradycardia are observed, it may be adequate to reduce the oxytocin dose by half or less when the FHR is normal, but there is abnormal uterine activity.

Figure 10.6a shows a reactive FHR at the beginning, but decelerations and tachycardia subsequently develop owing to increased frequency of contractions. In Figure 10.6b the FHR becomes tachycardic; towards the latter part of the trace, the dose of oxytocin was reduced to half and the tocographic transducer was adjusted. In Figure 10.6c the contractions have become less frequent, the FHR has settled to a normal baseline rate and is followed by a reactive pattern.

In cases of failure to progress in labour, oxytocin is commenced to augment uterine contractions. This may bring about FHR changes when the dose is increased to achieve the optimal target frequency of contractions. If the dose is reduced, the FHR pattern returns to normal but the uterine activity drops to suboptimal levels with no progress in labour. When FHR changes are encountered in such a situation, they may be transient and it may be worth stopping and re-starting oxytocin or reducing the dose. However, if abnormal FHR changes appear when oxytocin is recommenced despite these efforts, it may be better to deliver abdominally. In selected cases further time may be given to see whether the labour will progress without the use of oxytocin.

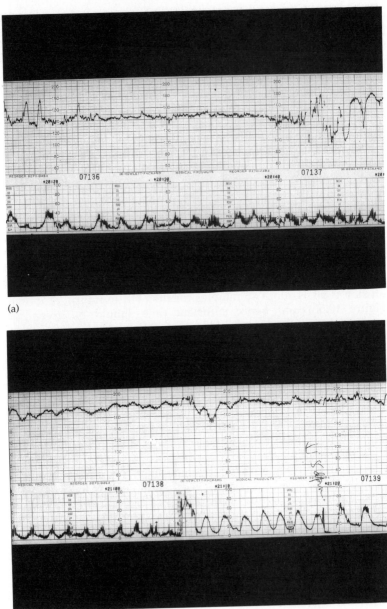

(a)

(b)

Figure 10.6   (a) Increased frequency of contractions: changes in trace; (b) sustained tachycardia; (c) reversion to normal after reduction of oxytocin

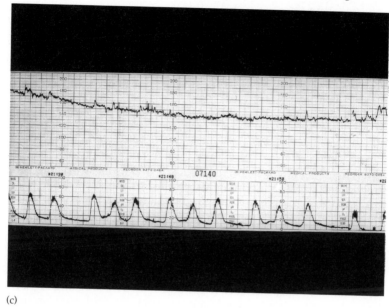

(c)

In induced labour, in the absence of disproportion, the uterus has to perform a certain amount of uterine activity depending on the parity and cervical score to achieve vaginal delivery. Considering this, it may be possible to achieve optimal uterine activity which does not cause FHR changes but is adequate to bring about slow but progressive cervical dilatation.[75] The labour may be a little longer, during which time adequate contractions are generated to achieve vaginal delivery. However, such management needs intrauterine catheters and equipment to compute uterine activity and it may not be possible to achieve optimal uterine activity without FHR changes and achieve vaginal delivery.

Chapter 11

Cardiotocographic interpretation: more difficult problems

Situations that are of specific concern and interest include prolonged bradycardia, placental abruption, sinusoidal pattern, the infected fetus, the abnormal fetus and the dying fetus.

Prolonged bradycardia

Prolonged fetal bradycardia (FHR <100 for 3 minutes or <80 for 2 minutes) is usually an acute event and may be a warning signal of acute hypoxia due to cord compression or prolapse, abruptio placentae, scar dehiscence, uterine hyperstimulation or another unknown cause. It can occur in healthy fetuses (possibly due to cord compression). Reversible causes for such an episode are epidural top-up, vaginal examination and uterine hyperstimulation. Simple measures such as adjusting maternal position, stopping the oxytocin infusion, attending to hydration and giving oxygen by face mask may correct the condition. A patient who presents with continuous abdominal pain, vaginal bleeding, a tender, tense or irritable uterus and prolonged fetal bradycardia is likely to have suffered an abruption and warrants immediate delivery. Those in whom scar dehiscence or rupture is suspected and those with cord prolapse may present with prolonged bradycardia and need immediate delivery. Most cases of prolonged bradycardia will show signs of recovery towards the baseline rate within 6 minutes. If the clinical picture does not suggest abruption, scar dehiscence or cord prolapse and if the fetus is appropriately grown at term with clear amniotic fluid and a reactive FHR pattern prior to the episode of bradycardia, return back to baseline FHR pattern within 9 minutes is to be expected. The recovery towards the normal baseline within 6 minutes with good baseline variability at the time of the bradycardia and during recovery are reassuring signs, and one should wait with confidence that the FHR will revert to the normal baseline with a normal pattern.

A 45-year-old multiparous woman was well known to the medical staff and midwives. A diagnosis of term labour was made at 22.00 hours when the cervix was 5 cm dilated and the initial CTG was normal (Figure 11.1a). Shortly before midnight a prolonged bradycardia became manifest after an otherwise normal trace (Figure 11.1b). The midwife correctly annotated 'FH' at the end of this strip of trace. Figure 11.1c shows the heart rate improving with good variability; however, the inexperienced obstetric registrar decided to perform a caesarean section and consequently the trace

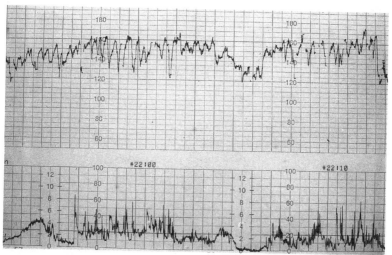

Figure 11.1   (a) CTG: normal reactive pattern

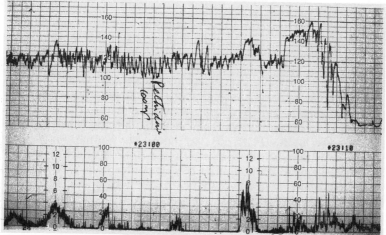

Figure 11.1   (b) Prolonged bradycardia

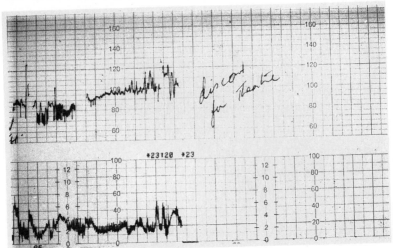

Figure 11.1   (c) Improvement in heart rate

shows 'discontinued for theatre'. Not surprisingly the Apgar scores were 9 at 1 minute and 10 at 5 minutes. If the trace had not been disconnected it would have reverted to normal; a premature decision led to an unnecessary caesarean section in a multiparous woman in whom labour was probably progressing rapidly. A longer contraction duration or transient cord compression might account for the deceleration. The diagnosis was obstetric registrar's distress!

If the FHR does not show signs of recovery by 9 minutes, the incidence of acidosis is increased, and one should take action to deliver the fetus as soon as possible.[82] The clinical picture has to be considered while anxiously awaiting the FHR to return to normal. Fetuses who are post-term, growth-restricted, have no amniotic fluid or have thick meconium-stained fluid at rupture of membranes are at a greater risk of developing hypoxia. Those with an abnormal or suspicious FHR trace prior to the episode of bradycardia are also at a greater risk of hypoxia developing within a short time. In these situations it may be better to take action early if the FHR fails to return to normal. If uterine hyperstimulation due to oxytocics is the cause, oxytocin infusion should be stopped. Inhibition of uterine contractions with a bolus intravenous dose of a beta-mimetic drug may be of value in some situations. Fetal scalp blood sampling (FBS) at the time of persistent prolonged bradycardia, or soon after, may delay urgently needed action. Figure 11.2 shows the trace in a case without obvious risk factors. Fetal scalp blood sampling, which

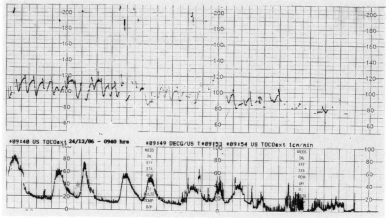

Figure 11.2   Fetal scalp blood sampling delays delivery: poor outcome

can prolong the bradycardia due to pressure on the fetal head, delayed delivery. Caesarean section was eventually performed. The baby had very poor Apgar scores and died on the third day after a period of neonatal convulsions.

Fetal acidosis observed soon after a bradycardia (Figure 11.3a) will recover when the trace returns to normal (Figure 11.3b). Alternatively, if the fetal heart does not return to normal, delivery should be undertaken. During a bradycardia the fetus reduces its cardiac output. Carbon dioxide and other metabolites cannot be cleared by the respiratory function of the placenta. The initial pH at the end of a bradycardia is low with a high $P\text{CO}_2$ showing a *respiratory acidosis*. Once the FHR returns to normal the carbon dioxide and metabolites are cleared, with the blood gases returning to normal in 30–40 minutes. If the episode of bradycardia continues then the fetus switches to anaerobic metabolism resulting in *metabolic acidosis* which is harmful to the fetus. Hence excessively prolonged bradycardia results in a poor outcome.

Scalp pH measurement should not be performed for prolonged bradycardia.

Scar rupture or dehiscence may not show the classical symptoms and signs of scar pain, tenderness, vaginal bleeding or alteration in maternal pulse or blood pressure. Changes in FHR or uterine activity may be an earlier manifestation of loss of integrity of the scar, and prompt action should avoid fetal or maternal morbidity or mortality. In these cases prolonged bradycardia may be an ominous sign and may indicate scar rupture. Figure 11.4a shows a prolonged bradycardia in a case of labour with a previous caesarean section.

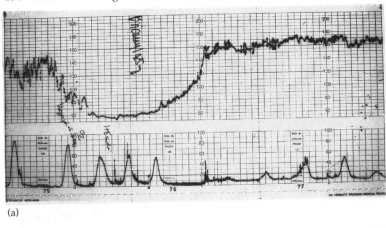

(a)

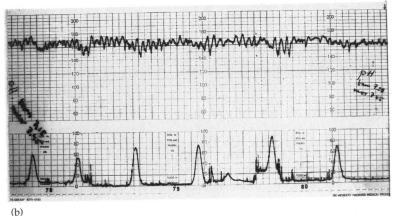

(b)

Figure 11.3   (a) Acidosis at time of bradycardia; (b) pH recovers after trace returns to normal

Delivery was delayed (Figure 11.4b), resulting in a baby with poor Apgar scores and neonatal asphyxial death on the second day. Whenever an operative delivery is planned the fetal heart should be checked prior to delivery as the baby may already be dead if there has been delay. In one such case prolonged bradycardia followed an eclamptic fit (Figure 11.5). The convulsions were controlled and the baby was delivered in 30 minutes: a reasonable delay to stabilize the maternal condition. The fetal heart was not verified just before delivery and the baby was a fresh stillbirth.[85] In cases of placental abruption it may not be possible to listen to the fetal heart with a

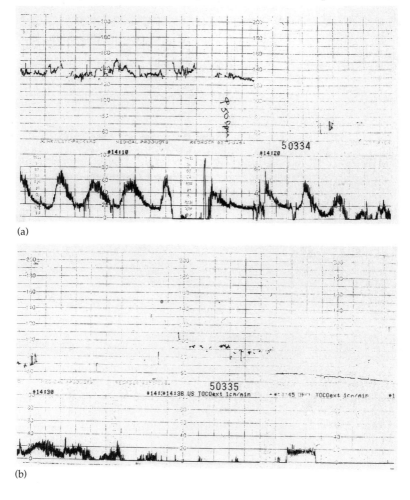

(a)

(b)

Figure 11.4 (a) Labour with previous caesarean section prolonged bradycardia; (b) delay in delivery leading to poor outcome

stethoscope or an electronic monitor. An ultrasound scan is therefore useful.

The procedure in the case of prolonged bradycardia is shown in Table 11.1. Each hospital should have facilities to perform an immediate caesarean section and deliver the baby within 15 minutes of taking the decision, especially if high-risk labours (such as cases of previous caesarean section) are being looked after.

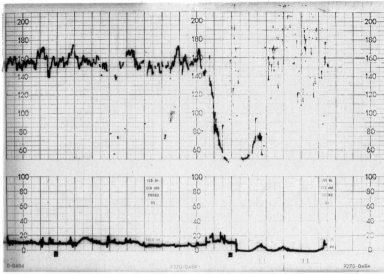

Figure 11.5   Prolonged bradycardia following eclamptic fit

Table 11.1   Procedure for prolonged bradycardia

3 minutes	Draw attention and review clinical picture and prior FHR trace
6 minutes	Expect recovery of FHR towards the baseline
9 minutes	If no recovery, prepare for operative delivery
12 minutes	Operative procedure should have started
15 minutes	Baby is delivered

Placental abruption

Figure 11.6 shows the initial trace in a woman having induction for proteinuric pregnancy-induced hypertension at term. The fundo-symphysis height was 36 cm at 40 weeks' gestation. Initially there is a slightly fast baseline rate with good variability but no accelerations (Figure 11.6a). A prostaglandin pessary was given and the initial contraction tracing is unremarkable. Forty minutes later the patient complained of increasing pain and restlessness. The toco-graphic tracing (Figure 11.6b) shows very frequent contractions of low amplitude which are typical of the irritable uterus in placental abruption. The FHR proceeded to a tachycardia with no further

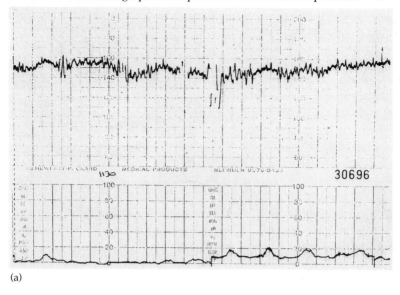

(a)

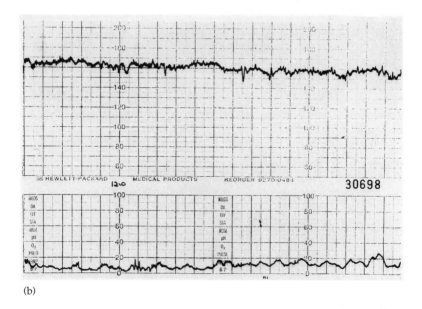

(b)

Figure 11.6   Induction for hypertension: (a) initial trace; (b) frequent
low-amplitude contractions, abnormal trace

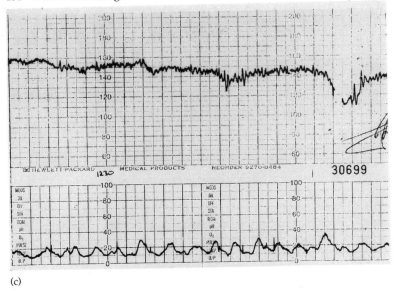

(c)

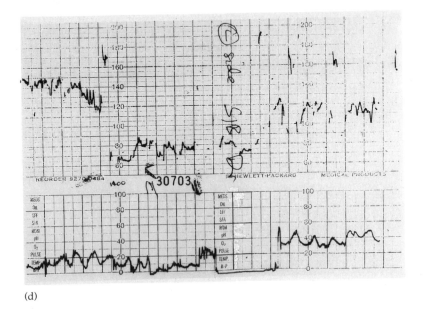

(d)

Figure 11.6   (c) Abnormal trace; (d) bradycardia

accelerations and with reduced baseline variability and a deceleration (Figure 11.6c). The woman suffered increasing pain, restlessness
and maternal tachycardia. There was no revealed bleeding; however, a clinical impression of placental abruption was clear. As the
woman was being prepared for caesarean section, the FHR dropped
abruptly to a bradycardia (Figure 11.6d). Immediate caesarean
section resulted in a moderately asphyxiated baby weighing 2.6 kg
who made a good recovery. There was a large retroplacental blood
clot.

**Frequent low-amplitude contractions and an abnormal CTG
trace suggest abruption.**

Sinusoidal FHR pattern

Sinusoidal FHR pattern is a description given to a trace with a
sinusoidal waveform appearance. Because of its association with
severe anaemia or hypoxic fetuses it is looked upon with anxiety. It
is important to realize that severely anaemic fetuses do not always
show sinusoidal pattern and that sinusoidal pattern can be
exhibited by healthy fetuses at certain times. A typical 'pathological'
sinusoidal FHR pattern should have a stable baseline rate of
110–150 bpm with regular oscillations having an amplitude of
5–15 bpm (rarely greater), a frequency of 2–5 cycles per minute and
a fixed or flat baseline variability.[86] Usually the oscillations of the
sinusoidal waveform above and below the baseline are equal.

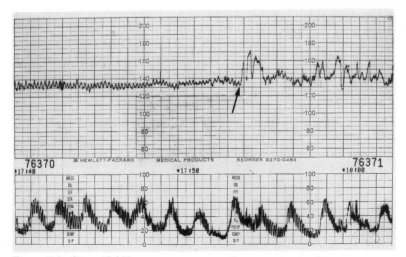

Figure 11.7   Sinusoidal-like trace: response to vibro-acoustic stimulus

However, the most important feature is that there are no areas of normal FHR variability and there are no accelerations. Rhythmic fetal mouth movements (observed by ultrasound) in a healthy fetus have been associated with 'physiological' sinusoidal FHR patterns. When encountered with such a pattern, stimulation of the fetus (e.g. vibro-acoustic) should produce accelerations of the FHR (Figure 11.7).[87] A fetus who is severely anaemic or hypoxic will not show accelerations, either spontaneously or in response to a stimulus (a child who is severely anaemic or hypoxic will not be able to throw a ball up and down and play). The neonatal outcome is the same in a fetus with spontaneous or sound-provoked accelerations observed on the FHR tracing. Reactivity and/or normal baseline variability in the FHR trace prior to or after the episode of a period of sinusoidal FHR pattern is suggestive of an uncompromised fetus. A 'saw-tooth' pattern of baseline variability instead of a smooth rounded sinusoidal wave-form might suggest it is not a 'pathological' sinusoidal FHR pattern. Figures 11.8 and 11.9 show typical sinusoidal FHR patterns, one in a fetus with a haemoglobin of 3 g/dl (0.47 mmol/l) due to Rhesus disease. When such a trace is encountered the possibility of Rhesus disease, anaemia due to other causes like infection, haemoglobinopathies (Bart's thalassaemia), fetomaternal transfusion or bleeding from the fetus (vasa praevia) should be considered. Relevant investigations such as testing for Rhesus antibodies, the Kleihauer-Betke test to detect fetal cells in the maternal blood, detection of thalassaemia carrier state or other appropriate investigations may be indicated.

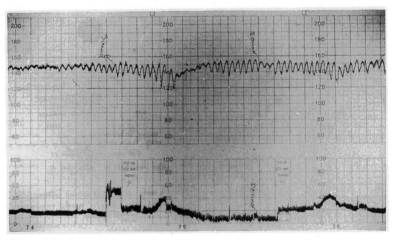

Figure 11.8   Sinusoidal pattern

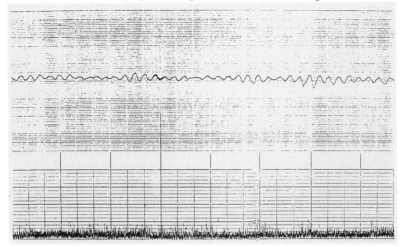

Figure 11.9   Sinusoidal pattern

At times sinusoidal heart rate patterns have been observed with the use of drugs like aphlaridine given to the mother.[88] Sometimes a typical sinusoidal pattern may not manifest and an atypical sinusoidal-like pattern may be seen in patients with fetal anaemia due to Rhesus disease or acute fetomaternal transfusion. Figure 11.10a shows a trace with most of the characteristics of sinusoidal pattern, but because of the absence of smooth sinus waveform and the unequal degree of oscillations above and below the baseline, the trace was not suspected to be abnormal and a decision was made not to consider this trace as sinusoidal in a growth-restricted fetus with no Rhesus disease. The trace was considered suspicious as there was no acceleratory response to sound. The NST repeated 3 days later showed an ominous pattern (Figure 11.10b). An immediate caesarean section was performed, and the baby had an Apgar score of 0, 0 and 3 at 1, 5 and 10 minutes respectively. The baby weighed 2.45 kg and had a haemoglobin level of 3.6 g/dl (0.56 mmol/l). The Kleihauer-Betke test on maternal blood was strongly positive, confirming a massive fetomaternal transfusion. The baby made a stormy recovery and subsequently developed cerebral palsy. 'Sinusoidal-like' traces are indicative of fetal anaemia[89,90] and can be recognized by familiarity with the typical pattern. Figure 11.11 shows another sinusoidal-like pattern due to fetomaternal transfusion.

Overdiagnosis of a sinusoidal trace without applying proper criteria is associated with normal outcome. Sinusoidal traces may be atypical with a poor outcome. Fetal blood sampling in labour to

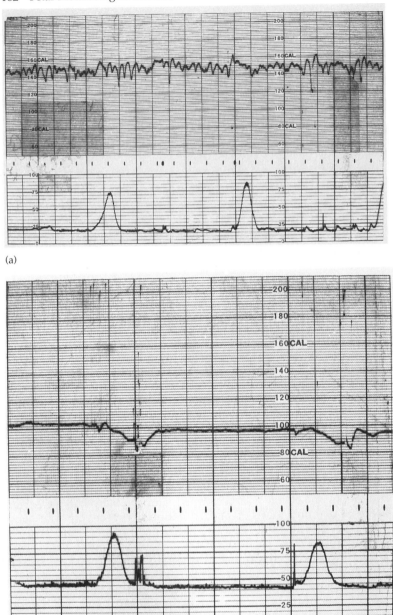

(a)

(b)

Figure 11.10   (a) Sinusoidal-like patterns: suspicious; (b) ominous pattern

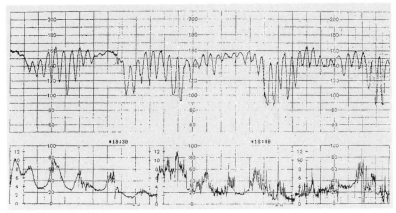

Figure 11.11 Sinusoidal-like pattern: fetomaternal transfusion

determine fetal haemoglobin level and fetal blood gases can be useful.

Fetal bleeding

An antepartum haemorrhage may rarely be due to fetal bleeding. This is a serious threat to the fetus because of its limited circulating blood volume. A woman was admitted with a small antepartum haemorrhage and a surprising CTG (Figure 11.12a). In most minor antepartum haemorrhages the CTG is normal because the bleeding is maternal blood and the placental circulation is not seriously threatened. In view of the CTG, induction of labour with continuous monitoring was undertaken. The CTG remained unusual (Figure 11.12b) but, in the absence of decelerations, we were confident there was no progressive hypoxia. At 15.25 h there was a fresh vaginal bleed with a dramatic change in the CTG to a saltatory, pseudo-sinusoidal picture (Figure 11.12c). This continued until delivery at 16.10 h (Figure 11.12d). Delivery was by caesarean section when vasa praevia was noted and the baby was found to be anaemic. The baby made a good recovery after blood transfusion.

Dramatic changes in the CTG with minor antepartum haemorrhage suggest vasa praevia.

The dying fetus

Fetal death is always preceded by a terminal bradycardia. The trace preceding this may show a variety of features, most commonly a tachycardia.

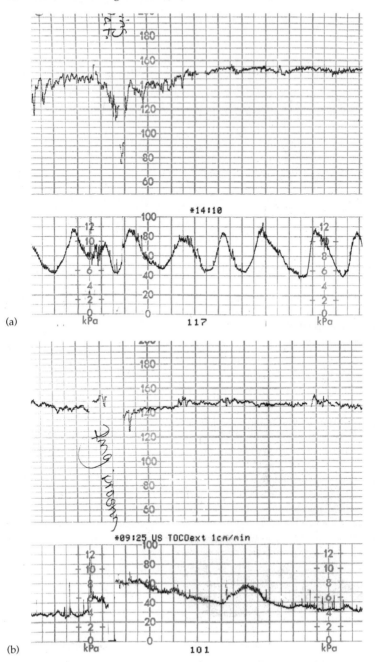

Figure 11.12   (a) CTG suscpicious therefore labour induced; (b) persistently abnormal CTG

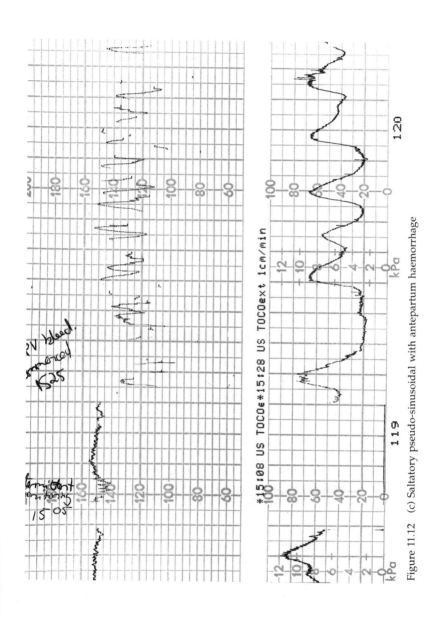

Figure 11.12   (c) Saltatory pseudo-sinusoidal with antepartum haemorrhage

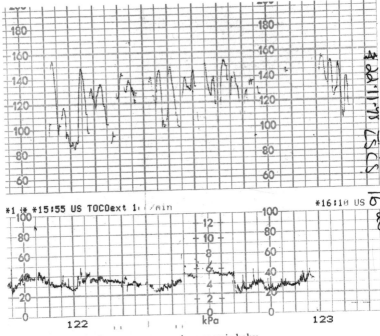

Figure 11.12   (d) Delivery: vasa praevia, anaemic baby

Figure 11.13 shows 10 sequential hourly traces in a mismanaged case of a high-risk mother suffering from sickle-cell disease. The baby was known to be small with oligohydramnios. For reasons difficult to comprehend the medical staff failed to act and at delivery this baby was in serious trouble. Severe variable decelerations are seen with a classical progression to tachycardia, absence of accelerations, reduced variability and terminal bradycardia. The baby was a fresh stillbirth. Knowing that the patient was a high-risk nulliparous woman, all who have read this book would have delivered the baby by the time of the third strip of tracing, when the baby would have been in reasonable condition. This high-risk woman had everything modern technology could offer, with the notable exception of basic common sense.

Some fetuses become so compromised in a more chronic way that they are unable to generate decelerations. This type of trace (Figures 11.14 and 11.15) is often misunderstood. There may be little in the way of a tachycardia but there is a complete absence of accelerations, a silent pattern of baseline variability and subtle shallow late decelerations. This is an ominous picture and the baby must be delivered.

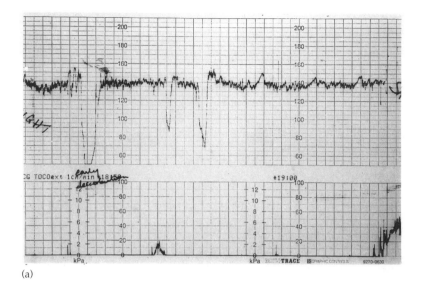

(a)

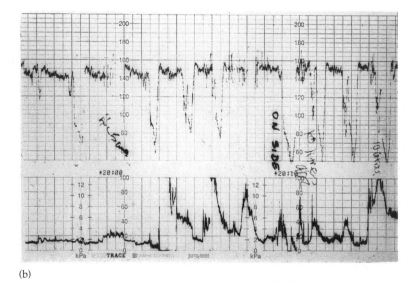

(b)

Figure 11.13 Dying fetus: (a) 1 hour; (b) 2 hours; (c) 3 hours; (d) 4 hours; (e) 5 hours; (f) 6 hours; (g) 7 hours; (h) 8 hours; (i) 9 hours; (j) 10 hours

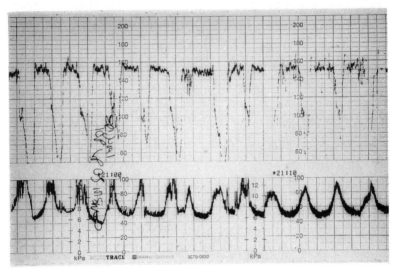

(c)

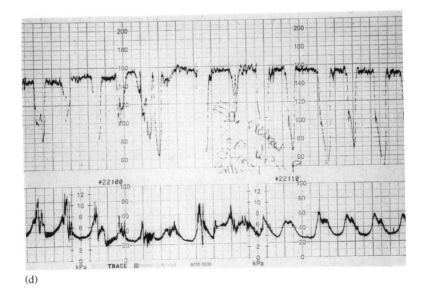

(d)

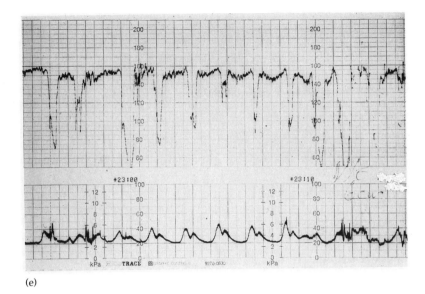

(e)

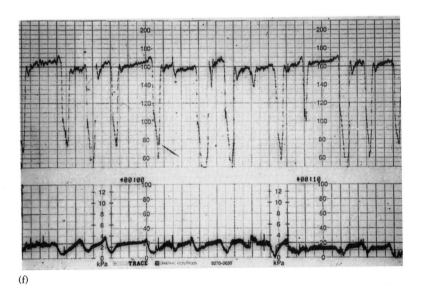

(f)

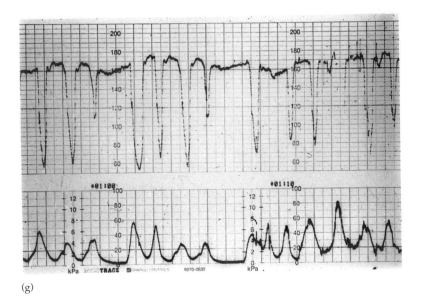

(g)

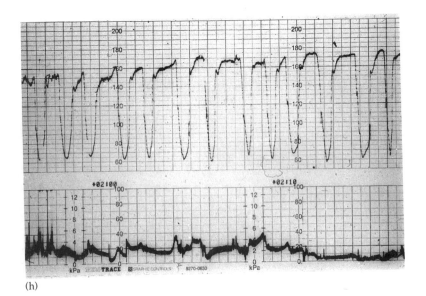

(h)

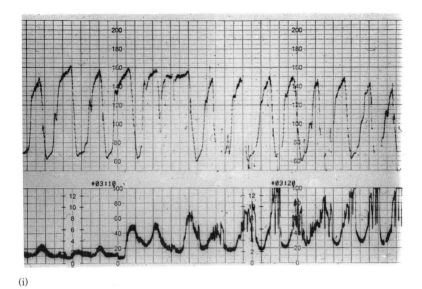

(i)

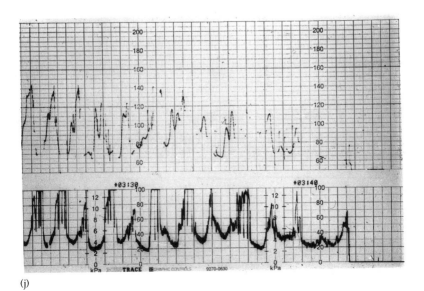

(j)

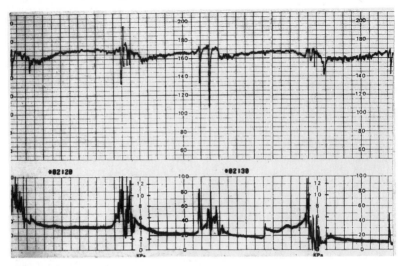

Figure 11.14   Ominous trace

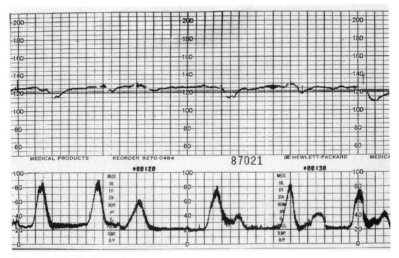

Figure 11.15   Ominous trace

An ominous tracing demands delivery.

Birth asphyxia is often associated with prelabour asphyxia. This highlights the value of the admission test. Should all babies with ominous traces be delivered with the expectation of a living, undamaged child? We are obliged to deliver all such babies but some features may indicate a poor prognosis.

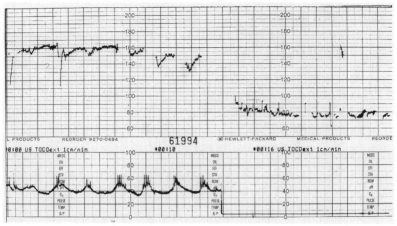

Figure 11.16 Terminal bradycardia

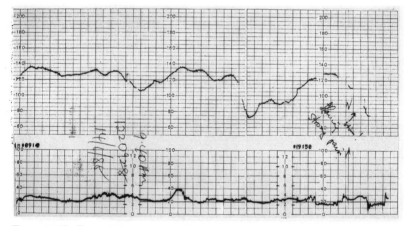

Figure 11.17 Terminal hypoxic central nervous system damage

A good trace within a reasonable period of the deterioration with an acute event such as an abruption suggests rapid intervention will be productive assuming a reasonable gestational age. Intervening when the main feature is tachycardia suggests some ability of the fetus to survive. Once the terminal bradycardia develops after the tachycardia the situation may be irretrievable (Figure 11.16), especially when there are features of a random, uncontrolled undulatory pattern with no baseline variability (Figure 11.17). This pattern suggests the possibility of central nervous system damage due to hypoxia. The challenge is to intervene in such pregnancies before this situation is reached; however, it should be kept in mind that central nervous system malformations can give rise to such patterns (see Chapter 6).

Chapter 12

The role of scalp pH

The availability of fetal scalp blood sampling for pH and its application in practice vary enormously. When the FHR is reactive and normal, the chance of fetal acidosis is extremely low.[91–93] On the other hand, suspicious and abnormal FHR changes are not always associated with acidosis.[92–95] Such observations form the basis of the perceived need to measure fetal scalp pH for further investigation.

Changes in the CTG cause anxiety to the person not familiar with CTG interpretation. An inexperienced person in a centre with fetal blood sampling (FBS) facilities might perform FBS more frequently. When properly interpreted, assessment of FHR changes in most cases proves of equal value to pH in predicting fetal outcome.[9] Fetal blood sampling is a useful adjunct because even with the worst pattern of tachycardia, reduced baseline variability and decelerations, only 50–60% of the fetuses are acidotic.[92] A wall chart correlating different FHR patterns to the percentage who are likely to be acidotic is available in most labour wards. It is clear from that chart and other studies that when the FHR pattern exhibited accelerations the chance of fetal acidosis was zero, emphasizing accelerations as the hallmark of fetal health.[92]

Baseline variability is another good indicator of fetal health. When normal baseline variability is observed in the last 20 minutes prior to delivery, the babies were in good condition at birth regardless of other features of the trace.[96] Fetal acidosis is more common when there is a loss of baseline variability with tachycardia or late decelerations.[92,97] The preservation of normal baseline variability indicates that the autonomic nervous system is responsive and the fetus is trying to compensate despite other abnormal features in the trace. The reason why even with a given FHR pattern there are different percentages of fetuses showing acidosis depends on the duration for which the suspicious or abnormal FHR pattern was present before the time of FBS.[10] The approximate duration after which acidosis develops in an appropriately grown term fetus with a given FHR pattern has been discussed previously. It is also known that in fetuses with less 'placental reserve' such as those with IUGR, thick, scanty meconium-stained fluid[98] and post-term infants, the rate of decline of pH is steep compared with term infants appropriately grown with abundant, clear amniotic fluid.

Respiratory and metabolic acidosis

Assessing pH alone does not suffice in identifying the fetus at risk and more comprehensive blood gas analysis may be necessary for clinical management. The placenta is the respiratory organ of the fetus. Reduction of perfusion of the placenta from the fetal vessels is manifest as variable decelerations due to cord compression and reduction of perfusion from the maternal circulation is represented by late decelerations. During the early stage of such threats the transfer of carbon dioxide from the fetal to maternal side is reduced leading to its accumulation. This results in respiratory acidosis manifested by a low pH and a high PCO_2. Respiratory acidosis is transitory particularly when corrective measures are taken and can be managed conservatively provided the FHR pattern improves. With a further reduction of perfusion from the maternal or fetal side the oxygen transfer becomes affected leading to anaerobic metabolism and metabolic acidosis in the fetus. This is manifested by a low pH, low PO_2 and low bicarbonate. Metabolic acidosis is damaging to the tissues. Transitory low pH values of respiratory type are not uncommon in low risk labours. Acidotic pH values in cord arterial blood and babies born with good Apgar scores are due to this phenomenon; 73% of babies with cord pH below 7.10 had a 1-minute Apgar score of more than 7 and 86% had a 5-minute Apgar score greater than 7.[99] These findings are probably due to respiratory acidosis which does not correlate well with fetal or neonatal condition. In this situation a comprehensive blood gas analysis including PCO_2, base excess and preferably lactic acid is desirable and more predictive. Caution should be exercised in using equipment that measures only pH. It is possible to determine the lactic acid level by the bedside with 20 μl of blood using the lactate card.[100]

Intrauterine infection with a high metabolic rate presents a greater oxygen demand to the fetus and metabolic acidosis might develop with minimal interruption of placental perfusion.

When to do FBS

Gradually developing hypoxia

The fetus becomes hypoxic and acidotic in labour in association with compromise of perfusion to the fetal or maternal side of the placental circulation. With the exception of situations of acute hypoxia due to cord prolapse, scar dehiscence, abruption and prolonged bradycardia it is unusual for a fetus that has shown accelerations and good baseline variability to become hypoxic without developing decelerations in labour. The decelerations indicate the presence of *stress* to the fetus whether from the challenge of poor perfusion or mechanical pressure. Provided the baseline fetal heart rate has not started to rise and there is no reduction in the baseline variability to less than 5 beats there is little to be gained by performing fetal blood sampling as the pH is likely to be normal. If the baseline FHR has risen by 20–30 beats and is not showing any further rise with a reduction in variability to less than 5 beats then *distress* is probable. Despite the fetus having increased its cardiac output to a possible maximum by increasing the fetal heart rate the functioning of the autonomic nervous system controlling the baseline variability is compromised by hypoxia. The time course of this process may be referred to as the *stress to distress period*. This period varies from fetus to fetus depending on the physiological reserve. This reserve is critically low in high risk situations of postmaturity, IUGR, intrauterine infection and in those with thick meconium and scanty amniotic fluid.

When the FHR shows hypoxic features suggestive of distress it is important to perform an FBS for pH and blood gases as the fetus may be or become acidotic. Initially this will be a respiratory followed by metabolic acidosis. Once the FHR shows a distress pattern, the time taken for metabolic acidosis to develop is unpredictable. After a certain duration of the distress pattern (*the distress period*) the FHR starts to decline in a rapid stepwise pattern culminating in terminal bradycardia and death (*the distress to death period*). The stress to distress interval (20.00 h–00.00 h, i.e. 4 h), the distress period (00.00 h–03.00 h, i.e. 3 h) and the distress to death period (03.00 h–03.40 h, i.e. 40 minutes) are illustrated by Figure 11.13 a–j. Another example where the stress to distress period, the distress period and the distress to death period are much shorter is shown in Figure 7.4 a–f. Clinical interpretation of FHR pattern will identify the onset of *stress*, *distress* and the *stress to distress period*. It will also identify the fetus in the *distress period*. An accurate prediction of the distress period cannot be made based on the FHR pattern as illustrated by the two examples. During the final decline phase (*distress to death period*), when the fetal heart rate drops irretrievably within a short period, it is often too late to intervene.

The value of FBS may be at the onset of the distress period and again repeated 30–40 minutes later or earlier depending on the baseline variability and the type of decelerations. The previous recommendation of immediate delivery when a pH is less than 7.20 (acidosis) and a repeat sample in 30 minutes or less when the pH is

7.20–7.25 (pre-acidosis) remains valid. Previous recommendations were that when the pH was greater than 7.25 repeat sampling was not required unless the FHR deteriorated. This approach may generate a false sense of security when the trace does not deteriorate although the pH is declining. The current FIGO recommendation is to repeat the pH in 30 minutes even when the first pH was in the normal range as this may indicate its rate of decline.[101] A decision for delivery can be made considering the rate of decline of the pH, the clinical risk factors (IUGR, thick meconium), parity, current cervical dilatation and rate of progress of labour.

Subacute hypoxia

The pH may deteriorate rapidly in a fetus who previously had a reactive trace without an increase in the baseline FHR if the decelerations are pronounced with large dip areas (drop of more than 60 beats for over 90 seconds) with the FHR recovering to the baseline only for short periods of time (less than 60 seconds). Examples of such traces are shown in Figure 12.1 a–f. In these situations a drop in pH can be by as much as 0.01 every 3–4 minutes. This decline in pH will be even steeper if the preceding trace was suspicious or abnormal or the clinical picture was one of high risk (IUGR, thick meconium with scanty fluid, or intrauterine infection). Further insults at this time, such as oxytocin infusion or a difficult instrumental delivery, may make the situation worse. With such traces attempts at FBS will delay much needed urgent delivery.

Chronic hypoxia

A non-reactive FHR pattern showing a baseline variability less than 5 beats with shallow decelerations (less than 15 beats for 15 seconds) even with a normal baseline rate indicates severe compromise and delivery should be expedited without delay to avoid fetal death (see Figure 7.6 a–d). A non-reactive trace with a baseline variability of less than 5 beats but without decelerations lasting more than 90 minutes indicates the possibility of already existing hypoxic compromise or damage due to other reasons (e.g. cerebral haemorrhage). This needs further evaluation if the pH is normal. In these circumstances fetal death may occur suddenly without further warning of a rise in baseline FHR or decelerations (see Figure 7.5 a–j). Hence, a non-reactive trace for greater than 90 minutes is abnormal and is an indication for further evaluation to rule out hypoxia.

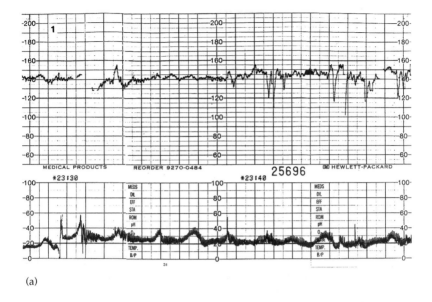

(a)

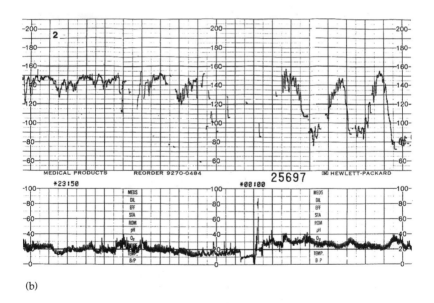

(b)

Figure 12.1   (a–f) Subacute hypoxia – prolonged decelerations (>90 seconds, depth >60 bpm) with short intervals of recovery (<60 seconds) to baseline rate

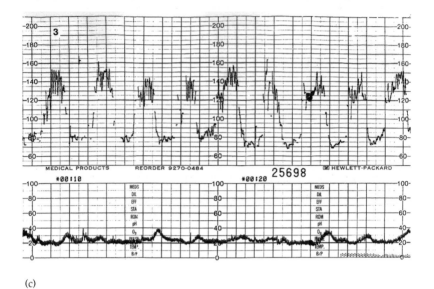

(c)

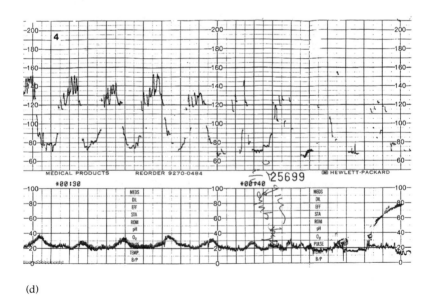

(d)

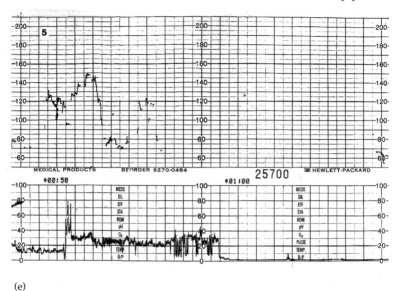

(e)

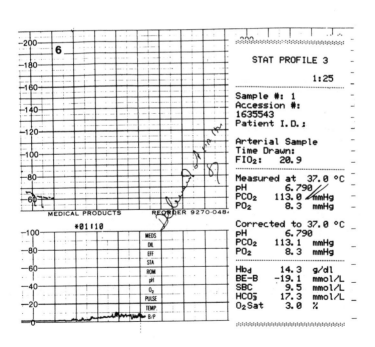

(f)

Acute hypoxia

Abruption, cord prolapse, scar dehiscence and uterine hyper-stimulation may give rise to acute hypoxia. This may manifest as prolonged bradycardia; at other times prolonged bradycardia occurs without obvious reason and in all circumstances is associated with rapidly progressive acidosis. With a bradycardia of less than 80 bpm the pH is likely to decline at the rate of approximately 0.01 per minute.[82]

With FHR patterns suggestive of acute or subacute hypoxia, performing FBS might delay intevention resulting in poor outcome. In FHR patterns with poor variability lasting for more than 90 minutes but with no decelerations, investigations should be performed to identify the cause. The principle can be established that the FHR pattern identifies the onset of stress (decelerations) and of distress (maximal elevation of baseline FHR with baseline variability less than 5 beats). Although the onset of stress and distress can be identified, the duration of the distress period before the fetus becomes hypoxic and acidotic cannot be predicted. A decision is required to deliver or to perform FBS, bearing in mind the clinical picture, if the prospect of early delivery is poor.

Alternative methods like ECG waveform analysis and pulse oximetry are being explored as primary modes of monitoring the fetus, but it is more likely they may have a place only in assisting clinical decision-making when the FHR shows a distress pattern. They may become an adjunct to FHR monitoring and may replace FBS. Computer-assisted interpretation of the CTG is likely to identify the onset of stress and distress but is unlikely to give an indication as to the duration of the distress period. The properly trained human brain is a very effective computer.

When not to do FBS

Frequently the FHR changes observed might be due to factors other than hypoxia. Dehydration, ketosis, maternal pyrexia and anxiety can give rise to fetal tachycardia but do not usually present with decelerations. Occipitoposterior position is known to be associated with more variable decelerations without hypoxic features evidenced by normal baseline rate and variability.[102] Oxytocin can cause hyperstimulation resulting in FHR changes of various forms which have been discussed in an earlier chapter. Prolonged bradycardia can be due to postural hypotension following epidural analgesia. Fetal heart rate changes should be correlated with the clinical picture before action is taken. In many instances remedial action such as hydration, repositioning of the mother or stopping the oxytocin infusion will relieve the FHR changes and no further action is necessary. When the FHR changes persist despite such action an FBS or one of the stimulation tests is warranted. At times FBS may not be necessary because the trace is reassuring, or it may show a low result transiently and later show a good result; the pH may be low transiently due to respiratory acidosis. Above all, when the trace is ominous or the clinical picture is poor it is better to deliver the baby rather than wasting time with FBS. At times a false reassurance leads to an unsatisfactory outcome. Fetal scalp blood sampling is often not appropriate under the following circumstances:

1 When the clinical picture demands early delivery (Figure 12.2): 42 weeks' gestation, cervix 3 cm dilated, thick meconium with scanty fluid.
2 When an ominous trace prompts immediate delivery (Figure 12.3).
3 When the FHR trace is reassuring (Figure 12.4).
4 When the changes are due to oxytocic overstimulation (see Figure 10.5).
5 When there is associated persistent failure to progress in labour (Figure 12.5).
6 During or soon after an episode of prolonged bradycardia (see Figure 10.4).
7 If spontaneous vaginal delivery is imminent or easy instrumental vaginal delivery is possible (see Figure 8.15).

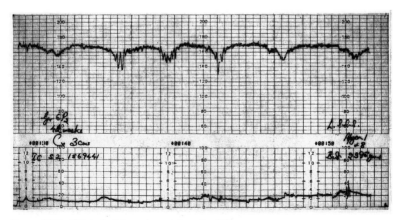

Figure 12.2   Clinical picture demands early delivery

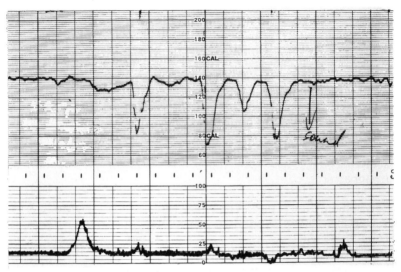

Figure 12.3   Ominous trace prompts immediate delivery

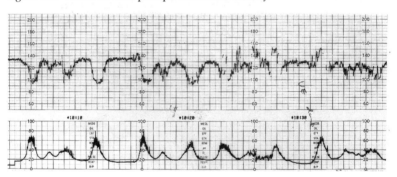

Figure 12.4   The FHR tracing is reassuring

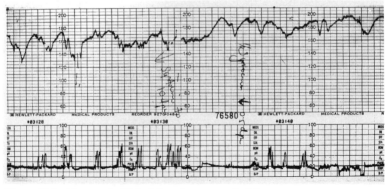

Figure 12.5   Changes in FHR: failure to progress in labour

Following these principles will help to avoid unnecessary FBS, operative deliveries and fetal morbidity from undue delay in delivery.

Alternatives to FBS

In practice FBS may not be performed because the facilities or the expertise are not available or because it is technically difficult. Alternative indirect methods are useful in this situation. A retrospective observation and correlation of the scalp blood pH to the presence or absence of accelerations at the time of FBS (Figure 12.6) led to the scalp stimulation test.[103] When the scalp was stimulated by pinching with a tissue forceps, if an acceleration was present it was unlikely that the scalp blood pH was below 7.20.[104,105] On the other hand, if there were no accelerations to such a stimulus only about 50% had acidotic pH values (<7.20), whereas a significant proportion had pre-acidotic values (7.20–7.25) and others had normal values (Table 12.1). Therefore this test was useful in identifying those who are not at risk, although it was not good in predicting those who are likely to be acidotic. In centres where facilities do not exist for scalp FBS, such a test would be a useful adjunct in reducing the number of unnecessary caesarean sections for 'fetal distress', and in centres where facilities are available for FBS, it will reduce the number of samples taken. Where there is a failure to obtain a sample during the FBS procedure, observation of

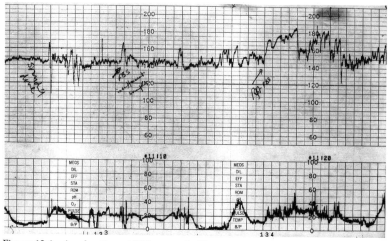

Figure 12.6   Acceleration at FBS, normal pH

Table 12.1   Results of scalp stimulation tests in relation to scalp blood pH values[103–105]

Response to scalp stimulation	Fetal scalp blood pH values			Total
	<7.20	7.20–7.25	>7.25	
	n = 82	n = 156	n = 462	n = 700
Positive response	1 (0.4%)	33 (12.7%)	226 (86.9%)	260
Negative response	40 (44.4%)	45 (50.0%)	5 (5.6%)	90
Total	41 (11.7%)	78 (22.3%)	231 (66%)	350

an acceleration is very reassuring and the procedure can be discontinued.

In the study described above, the case that recorded a positive response with an acidotic pH showed respiratory acidosis, which is due to accumulation of CO_2, is not harmful to the fetus and is known to reverse itself once the FHR returns to normal. Careful observation of the characteristics of the FHR resulted in a fetus born with good Apgar scores. An alternative to the scalp stimulation test is a fetal acoustic stimulation test (FAST) in labour (Figure 12.7).[106] There were a number of reports from the USA showing the fetus responding with FHR acceleration to FAST if it was not acidotic. Although the majority of fetuses with non-acidotic pH responded

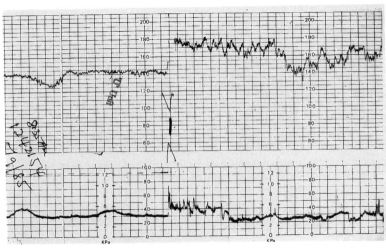

Figure 12.7   Accelerative response to vibro-acoustic stimulus

with acceleration, when they failed to respond only about 50% had acidotic pH values, which was similar to the results of the scalp stimulation test. It is difficult to explain why the fetal response of acceleration should be associated with arbitrary cut-off points of scalp blood pH values; however, it is known that auditory sensation is one of the first to be affected by hypoxia and negative response to acoustic stimulation might warn of the possibility of hypoxia. Fetal acoustic stimulation is a new modality used to test fetal well-being and concern has been raised about safety aspects. Studies performed on its safety have shown that there is no evidence of catecholamine release with the stimulus,[107] no hearing loss[108] and no long-term disturbance to the fetal behavioural state studied by FHR variability cycles.[109] With these alternative methods available there is a tendency for physicians to perform FBS less frequently, and even a willingness to replace this test by FAST or scalp stimulation tests.[110] Care should be exercised if relying on such stimulation tests alone, because 50% of fetuses who do not show a reaction to the FAST or scalp stimulation have non-acidotic pH values, and some fetuses show a positive response even with acidotic pH values (Figure 12.8).[111,112]

The Royal College of Obstetricians and Gynaecologists Study Group has recommended that fetal scalp blood sampling facilities should be available in any hospital where electronic fetal monitoring is performed.[113] However, clinicians who understand the

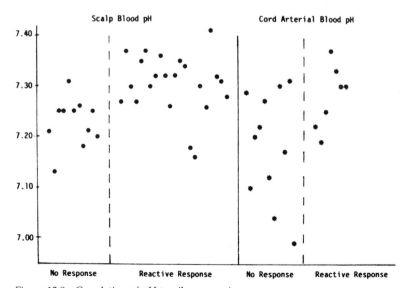

Figure 12.8   Correlation of pH to vibro-acoustic response

clinical situation and the fetal heart rate pattern may make a decision without resorting to fetal blood sampling and without an increase in caesarean section rate for fetal distress.[110] In many situations it may be wiser to proceed to delivery without wasting precious time. It has been shown that if the decision-to-delivery interval in situations of fetal distress is 35 minutes as opposed to 15 minutes the admission rate to the neonatal intensive care unit is doubled.[114] FBS is not always possible because facilities may not be available or it may be difficult to perform due to an undilated cervix or high head.[115,116] In these situations decisions based on the CTG and the clinical situation remain critical.

Chapter 13

Alternative methods of intrapartum fetal surveillance

Despite the limited contribution of birth asphyxia to cerebral palsy and doubts cast on the benefits of intrapartum electronic fetal monitoring, research is in progress to find better methods of monitoring to avoid the tragedies which can occur due to birth asphyxia. Every now and then such tragedies are highlighted by litigation and the large awards of damages. There is little doubt that the practice of intrapartum fetal monitoring is likely to stay, but whether it will be in the form of electronic fetal heart rate monitoring or by other means, or by a combination, is difficult to predict. This chapter reviews why there is a search for newer methods, some of the newer methods available and what may happen in the future.

Why is there a search for new methods?

There are problems in correlating the FHR changes with fetal acidosis. When the trace is normal, the chances of fetal acidosis are small, but when changes occur, only up to 50% or fewer are noted to be acidotic.[92] This is because a fetus does not become acidotic with the onset of FHR changes. Depending on the physiological reserve, one fetus may react differently from another to the hypoxic insult. It has been observed that for 50% of averagely-grown term fetuses with clear amniotic fluid and a reactive trace, it takes 115 minutes with repetitive late decelerations, 145 minutes with repetitive variable decelerations and 185 minutes with a flat trace for it to become acidotic from the onset of the abnormality of the trace, which implies that some may become acidotic in a shorter period of time.[10] This duration may be even shorter when there is reduced physiological reserve as may be the case in post-term and growth-retarded fetuses and in those with scanty, thick meconium-stained fluid. Therefore, it becomes necessary for FHR changes to be verified by fetal scalp blood sampling (FBS) to identify those with acidosis in order to avoid increasing the caesarean section rate. However, facilities and expertise are not available to perform FBS in many centres,[115,116] and its value is questioned by some.[110] These problems have prompted research into newer methods of fetal surveillance in labour.

Fetal ECG waveform analysis

The concept of ECG waveform analysis as a method of fetal monitoring is not new. Changes in the ST segment of the fetal ECG are related to metabolic events in the fetal myocardium during hypoxia, and changes in time constants, like the PR or RR intervals (fetal heart rate), suggest neurophysiological responses to hypoxia. These two functions are largely independent but with a significant overlap. Additional information may be gained when the fetal heart rate and T/QRS ratio are studied. Previous attempts to elucidate the role of ST waveform analysis during labour have provided conflicting evidence. In retrospect, there appear to be several reasons for this. The main reason is the use of filters to reduce the signal to noise ratio which attenuates the ECG waveform changes. On the basis of experimental data together with developments in bioengineering, advances have been made in the last few years resulting in production of the STAN-ST analyser (Cinventa AB, Molndal, Sweden) to analyse ST waveform in labour.

Experimental data have suggested that the appearance of high peaked T waves together with an elevation of the ST segment signifies an imbalance of the myocardial energy situation with anaerobic metabolism and glycogenolysis. This important defence mechanism is known to operate with an increase in circulating catecholamine (β-adrenoceptor stimulation);[117] this brings about a shift in K^+ which increases the T-wave amplitude (Figure 13.1). A T/QRS ratio less than 0.25 is regarded as the upper level of normality based on the reported mean T/QRS ratio of 0.148 with a standard deviation of 0.048 in normal fetuses during labour.[118] Based on earlier data and a multicentre study on human fetuses, the 0.5 level signifies a hypoxia. This evolving hypoxic state showing a rise in the T/QRS ratio with an abnormal FHR pattern can be recorded without much difficulty (Figure 13.2). Each fetus has a steady level of T/QRS ratio throughout the first stage of labour and could be identified from the initial recording. It is possible to record the FHR pattern, the ECG complex with T/QRS analysis and uterine contractions in one trace (Figure 13.3). Although initial results were promising,[119] a further study trying to correlate FHR changes, fetal scalp blood pH and umbilical arterial acid–base values failed to show correlation between the development of acidosis and fetal ECG changes.[120] A randomized study consisting of nearly 500 subjects has shown a reduction in the caesarean section rate when

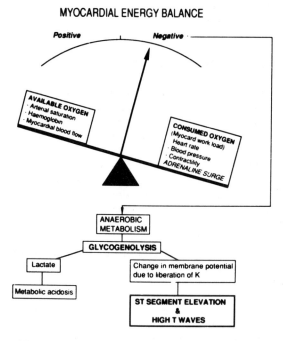

Figure 13.1   ECG waveform changes: pathophysiological mechanism

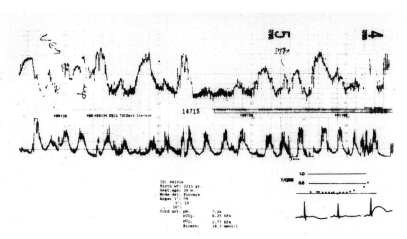

Figure 13.2   Raised T/QRS ratio with abnormal CTG

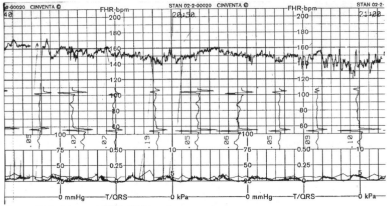

Figure 13.3   Trace of FHR, ECG and contractions

the ECG waveform analysis was used in conjunction with CTG compared with CTG alone.[121] This work requires confirmation by other studies.

One of the problems in evaluating this modality was the difficulty of monitoring perinatal asphyxia prospectively because of the low true incidence of asphyxia and because of interference based on existing methods of fetal surveillance. Studies are limited in numbers because of the above factors and the results of a large European multicentre study are awaited. In the meantime this technique should only be applied within the context of research studies.

Systolic time intervals of the fetal cardiac cycle

Laboratory and clinical studies have suggested that the systolic time intervals (STIs) of the cardiac cycle may be sensitive indicators of cardiac function and fetal compromise. The main STIs are the pre-ejection period (PEP) from the onset of ventricular depolarization to the opening of the aortic valve, and the ventricular ejection time (VET) from the aortic opening to aortic closure. The PEP is an indicator of myocardial contractility and the VET mainly reflects peripheral resistance.

The QRS complex of the fetal heart, derived in labour by scalp electrode, provides an easily obtainable and identifiable signal of ventricular polarization. The precise and consistent identification of aortic valvular events is difficult. The most satisfactory available technique relies on Doppler ultrasound for the detection of cardiac motion. The detection of individual valvular events is effected by a series of time and amplitude gates. The signals that pass through these gates are regenerated to provide precise indications of the timing of mitral valve closure, aortic valve opening and closure, and mitral valve opening. Similar signals are derived from the fetal electrocardiogram. From these signals, the intervals can be determined electronically. The digital measurements of time can then be converted to analogue form for recording alongside uterine activity and fetal heart rate on a strip chart recorder. In pregnancy, STIs are affected by many factors besides myocardial compromise, including heart rate, gestational age, birth weight, cardiac preload and afterload, hypoxia and acidosis.[122] From animal and adult studies it is known that STIs can also be affected by peripheral resistance, inotropic drugs, valvular disease, and cardiac arrhythmias.[123] Fetal STIs have been studied for changes associated with FHR patterns during labour. Periodic accelerations are associated with prolongation of PEP and shortening of VET. Early decelerations are associated with a mild prolongation of periodic PEP,[124] and a slight prolongation of the VET, inversely proportional to the FHR.[125] Variable decelerations are associated with prolonged periodic PEP values. Changes in VET are variable and prolonged VETs were seen with severe decelerations because of the inverse relationship with fetal heart rate. The relationship between STI changes and late decelerations is not clear and is probably dependent on whether fetal hypoxia is acute or chronic, and the presence of acidosis. It is likely that shortening of baseline PEP occurs with late decelerations in early stages, while prolongation of PEP, reflecting myocardial depression, occurs with severe (hypoxic) late decelerations and acidosis. During labour, STIs may prove to be of value in elucidating equivocal fetal heart rate patterns, and in detecting fetal hypoxia and acidosis. A shortening of the baseline PEP between contractions may reflect the onset and progression of hypoxia. However, technical improvements are required together with further clinical studies comparing STI measurements with current monitoring techniques to define the sensitivity and specificity.

Pulse oximetry

Modern monitoring of anaesthetic and neonatal patients includes pulse oximetry. Pulse oximeters are cheap and non-invasive, and monitor both heart rate and arterial oxygen saturation (Sao_2). The accuracy of the method has been established and, unlike Pao_2 monitors, pulse oximeters respond rapidly to changes in the oxygen content in the blood. There are specific advantages of recording Sao_2 instead of partial pressure of oxygen (Pao_2). The oxygen pressure electrode requires frequent calibration. It necessitates shaving hair and firm fixation techniques. The relation of oxygen saturation and partial pressure is defined by the oxygen dissociation curve, and a small change in Pao_2 is represented by a large change in Sao_2; large changes are easier to detect and are less affected by technical errors. An increase in hydrogen ion concentration or 2,3-diphospho-glycerate shifts the oxygen dissociation curve to the right; a baby who is acute or chronically hypoxaemic and/or acidaemic may have a normal Pao_2 but its oxygen saturation will be low. However, obvious disadvantages exist with the use of pulse oximetry in labour. The cervix must be open enough to insert the probe. Intact membranes, however, are not a contraindication to pulse oximetry – in fact, amniochorionic membranes do not affect oximetry readings. Oxygen saturation readings are affected in fetuses developing palpable caput formation and when meconium staining of the amniotic ·fluid is seen. Pulse oximetry is unsuitable in cases of preterm labour, antepartum haemorrhage or twins. It is also difficult to obtain good recordings in fetuses with thick, curly hair.

Fetal monitoring with pulse oximetry has been studied.[126] Pulse oximetry was successful in 86 of 145 (60%) patients in labour. Fifty-one were recorded in early labour (cervical dilatation <5 cm) with a mean oximetry reading of 68% (range 11–81%). Twelve patients were recorded in mid-labour (cervix 6–8 cm) with a mean oximetry reading of 60% (range 40–80%). In late labour (cervix > 9 cm dilatation), the mean oximetry reading was 58% (range 29–80%). This means that the oxygen saturation gradually fell with the progress of labour. The largest range of decline in oximetry reading from a labour that was initially uncomplicated was from 81% to 11%. In that patient severe cardiotocographic decelerations accompanied the drop in oxygen saturation; the patient was delivered by lower segment caesarean section and a loop of the cord was found by the baby's ear.

The oximetry values of 68% in healthy fetuses during early labour and a value of 58% before birth are higher than values derived from pH and Pao_2 in the literature. As deoxygenated blood in the inferior vena cava mixes with oxygenated blood from the umbilical vein, scalp oximetry readings should be below values in the umbilical vein. However, pulse oximeters are empirically calibrated using a calibration curve constructed from transmission probes on healthy adults over an oxygen saturation range of 70–100%. The oximeter's microprocessor unjustifiably extrapolates the curve at lower levels of saturation and therefore reflectance readings from the fetus will need small calibration adjustments to take into account fetal haemoglobin concentration, reflectance techniques and the low oxygen levels. Irrespective of all these considerations, a change in oximetry reading will still reflect a change in fetal oxygenation.

The fetal pulse oximetry technique is limited by caput, fetal hair, a wide normal range, poor calibration and difficulties in registering signals. Before pulse oximetry can be used in clinical practice, further development of the method is necessary.

Doppler ultrasound

The benefit of Doppler umbilical artery blood flow recording as a tool for antenatal assessment of fetal well-being in high-risk pregnancies has been documented in several studies.[127,128] A semiquantitive blood flow class system describing blood velocity waveform with emphasis on the end-diastolic part was the most powerful marker of imminent fetal asphyxia and of intrauterine growth restriction. In experimental asphyxia in fetal lambs, aortic mean blood flow velocities were reduced. Aortic blood flow waveforms showed low end-diastolic flow velocities and/or increased pulsatility indices (PI).[129] In the common carotid artery of the fetuses, the PI tended to decrease during asphyxia and the umbilical artery PI remained unchanged. The changes in the fetal aortic velocity waveforms indicate an adaptation of the peripheral circulation to asphyxia. The waveform changes seem to be a late phenomenon in the process of asphyxia.

Doppler ultrasound of the umbilical artery flow velocity waveform was studied prospectively as an admission test at the labour ward in 575 women in various stages of labour before, during and after uterine contractions, and evaluated in relation to intrapartum and fetal outcome variables.[51] Fetuses who are small for gestational age had significantly more abnormal blood flow velocity waveforms than did fetuses who were appropriate for gestational age, and more patients with umbilical artery acidaemia had abnormal blood flow velocity waveforms compared with those with normal pH. However, no association was found between abnormal flow velocity waveforms and cord complications, meconium-stained amniotic fluid or abnormal fetal heart rate tracing, nor was there any association with operative delivery for fetal distress or low Apgar scores at 1 minute and 5 minutes. Doppler recording of the umbilical artery flow velocity waveform as an admission test at the labour ward was not a good predictor of fetal distress.

A patient with a small-for-gestational-age fetus at 36 weeks had a non-stress test (NST) that showed a non-reactive trace. However, the umbilical artery Doppler velocity waveform showed normal blood flow (Figure 13.4). Because of the clinical picture (FSH of 30 cm at 36 weeks and clinically reduced amniotic fluid) and a non-reactive NST, labour was induced. The cervix was 1 cm long and 1 cm dilated. On rupture of membranes there was scanty but clear

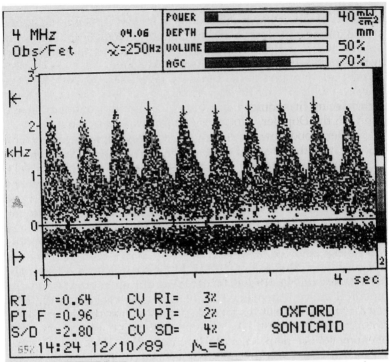

Figure 13.4   Doppler blood flow velocity waveform in the umbilical artery of a growth-restricted fetus at term

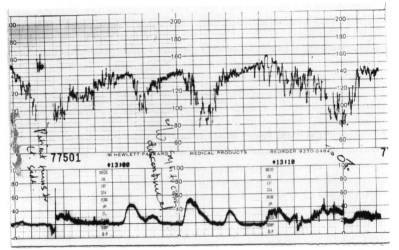

Figure 13.5   Trace of growth-restricted fetus with normal Doppler results showing variable and late decelerations with commencement of oxytocin for induction of labour

amniotic fluid. With 2.5 mU/minute of oxytocin, contractions of one in 2–3 minutes occurred and with each contraction there were variable to late decelerations (Figure 13.5). The baby was delivered by caesarean section, weighed 1.8 kg and had an Apgar score of 9 at both 1 and 5 minutes and a cord arterial pH of 7.28. Although the baby was in good condition, with a given clinical picture and the FHR tracing it would have been unwise to continue labour, although the Doppler velocity waveform was reassuring.

Doppler blood flow measurements in labour appear to be useful in evaluating the effects of drugs on uterine and fetal blood flow in labour, but have little to contribute to routine intrapartum fetal monitoring. Sophisticated equipment as well as trained personnel are needed to perform good measurements, making this method difficult to implement in a continuous form or even as an intermittent method in labour.

Continuous pH measurements

Much effort has been expended over many years to develop a continuous pH electrode and to perform continuous pH measurements in labour. This has been fraught with technical difficulties. The electrodes tend to be large, difficult to apply and fragile. Furthermore, there appears to be a drift in the value when the electrode is in place over a long period of time. Caput formation and venous stasis can affect the readings. It is not uncommon to find occasional low pH of a respiratory type in a healthy baby during labour which tends to recover on its own with passage of time. In studies dealing with pH in labour the mean pH is calculated from a large number of fetuses. The mean acid–base values from 130 cases of low risk labour are given in Table 13.1.[130]

Table 13.1 Acid–base values in scalp and cord blood (mean value)

	Cervical dilatation		
	5 cm	10 cm	Cord arterial blood
pH	7.332	7.335	7.292
P_{CO_2}	66.85	66.87	50.56
P_{O_2}	25.00	24.06	21.05
HCO_3	24.15	23.93	23.08

Table 13.2   Distribution of pH values in scalp and cord blood

pH	Cervical dilatation				Cord arterial blood	
	5 cm		10 cm			
	n	%	n	%	n	%
<7.10	–	–	–	–	2	1.7
<7.15	1	0.8	2	1.7	4	3.4
<7.20	2	1.7	3	2.5	9	7.5
<7.25	7	5.8	7	5.8	31	25.8
<7.30	31	25.8	28	23.7	61	50.8
>7.30	89	74.8	90	76.3	59	49.2

In this series there were individual cases with low pH values (Table 13.2), but since the FHR recordings were satisfactory labour was allowed to progress and the babies were delivered vaginally. At delivery the Apgar scores were good and the cord pH values were not acidotic, indicating that transient changes in pH are not an uncommon finding in any labour; these changes are mostly of a respiratory type and will correct themselves with time.

From a large series in the UK[99] it was reported that 73% of infants with cord arterial pH below 7.10 had a 1-minute Apgar score of over 7 and 86% had a 5-minute Apgar score over 7. Low arterial pH is usually due to accumulation of carbon dioxide and its influence on pH. Respiratory acidosis is poorly correlated with fetal or neonatal condition. Clearly, it would be difficult to manage patients on continuous pH measurements alone, and additional information on the blood gases is required. Information from the FHR pattern along with continuous pH measurements may improve the present standards of intrapartum fetal surveillance.

Any new method of fetal surveillance generates great enthusiasm when first applied. Caution must be exercised before wider clinical implementation. Full studies and trials are mandatory. It should be recognized that new methods may involve greater invasion and inconvenience for the woman.

Chapter 14

Computers and the cardiotocograph

Modern technology may be applied to the CTG to aid its display and transmission, to store data and to assist in decision-making. Most manufacturers now offer sophisticated electronic systems. Central station displays which allow overviewing of all monitors in the labour ward and selective display of any individual monitor are available. There are two problems with this attractive technology. Midwives traditionally provide bedside care and a central display might inhibit this. These displays incorporate alert and alarm signals, which can be set at particular levels locally; however, experience shows that the variety of fetal heart rate patterns seen does not lend itself easily to such a framework. It is common for midwives and doctors to use such devices initially but later to turn them off. The distant transmission of a CTG over a telephone system may be appropriate in some areas where distances are great, and can be a way to obtain second opinions. We must remember, however, that although we all enjoy playing with toys, novelty value is never a justification for technology: it must be shown to improve the care provided. The technology is available to record the CTG on earth of a pregnant woman on the moon if she went there!

Data management, storage, retrieval and archiving represent a much stronger justification for the application of this technology. Problems arising from obstetric practice head the list in the medical litigation scene in most countries. Analysis of the problems indicates that many of these cases concern the management of labour and fetal monitoring. It is not only misjudgment or lack of knowledge which has caused this; one of the factors contributing appears to be the failure of documentation of events in labour. It is important to document the date and time of each event in labour and the interrelationship of FHR pattern to vaginal examination findings, administration of drugs and other episodes. To facilitate this the manufacturers of fetal monitors have produced equipment that self-annotates the FHR trace with the date, time and mode of recording (e.g. ultrasound, fetal ECG, external or internal tocograph). A key pad or a bar-coded entry system can be attached to the fetal monitor to enable additional findings such as results of a vaginal examination, colour of amniotic fluid, etc. to be entered on the trace. Not only are the entered data printed on the trace but they are registered in the mother's obstetric notes which are maintained in the computer (with date and time of entry). This can be reviewed from time to time, updated or printed to obtain a hard copy. Based on the cervical examination findings entered by the bedside via the keypad of the fetal monitor, a partogram may be automatically drawn on the computer screen. These obstetric management systems not only keep the most wanted records but will also form a reserve for future research and to generate statistics. Most systems can keep up to 8 hours of labour record notes and the FHR tracing of 4000 subjects in a small optical disc which can be kept for many years. Tampering with the records on a subsequent occasion is impossible. Though a costly investment, in the long run it will pay for itself even if it helps to solve only one medico-legal case in which the records have been lost using traditional record-keeping.

Can computers assist in decision-making? Data may be processed to provide indices of the fetal heart rate other than those previously discussed. The Oxford Sonicaid System 8000 performs this function on antenatal fetal heart rate recordings. It provides a screen display of the CTG and also stores every trace recorded on a hard drive. This information can be recalled at short notice and provides a valuable system for research studies. The analysis system programmed by Dawes and Redman assesses various features of the tracing, defining accelerations as a rise in baseline of 10 beats for 10 seconds and assessing baseline variability as mean range.[131] Mean range of variation is considered the most important index: if it is greater than 20 milliseconds it is normal. The information produced is highlighted as 'advisory only' and clinical decisions remain the responsibility of the clinician. Such programmes may have some value educationally and for research purposes; however, there is a danger they may be seen as a short cut to interpreting the CTG without proper understanding. The further danger is that staff will lose their skills in intrapartum CTG interpretation which cannot be subjected to the same computerized analysis. A comparison was made between the value given as a score between 1 and 100 by an experienced observer for a series of antenatal CTGs and the Dawes Redman score. There was a wide degree of agreement and a very strong correlation.[132]

Attempts have been made to devise a computer system to aid the interpretation of intrapartum CTGs. The problem has been the great variability of pattern of fetal heart rate depending on both physiological and pathological mechanisms. In addition the CTG cannot be separated from the clinical scenario. A multicentre study was performed comparing the opinion of 17 experts with the analysis of an intelligent computer system for managing labour using the CTG.[133] The system's performance was found to be indistinguishable from the experts' in the 50 cases examined, but it was more consistent. This demonstrates the potential for an intelligent computer system to improve the interpretation of the CTG and decrease intervention. Furthermore, the good performance of most experts in this study demonstrates the potential effectiveness of the CTG and raises important questions regarding why the CTG has fallen short of expectations in current practice.

The best computer is the one most freely available in all labour wards: the human brain.

Chapter 15

Medico-legal issues

Many doctors and midwives are anxious about medico-legal action and complaints. This is understandable; however, certain logical steps can be taken to manage the risk.

We should try to understand why families take legal action and the nature of this action. It most often relates to a damaged child. Although financial support is part of the objective, every family would rather have a healthy child. The legal process itself is long and tedious. The family would much rather devote the precious time in looking after the injured child. The families often feel that they have not been given an explanation of what happened and communication has been poor. They also feel that what has happened to them should not happen to other people.

The legal process involves establishing liability and causation.

Liability

So far as damage to a child is concerned, the time lapse before the commencement of litigation is unlimited. The child's claim is made by the mother or father (next friend) on behalf of the child. If the claim relates to damage to the mother then a limitation of 3 years applies.

The mother makes a statement as to what she believes happened or did not happen related to the damage which she alleges. A solicitor then conducts the legal process. The clinical notes are requested from the hospital. These will be (have to be) exactly as compiled by the staff at the time. The importance of careful, legible note keeping is obvious. Regrettably, in many hospitals the standard is poor. Midwives in general keep very good notes. Junior doctors more often than not have illegible signatures and may not date and time their entry to the notes. At every interaction between a doctor and the mother an entry must be made. This should preferably be by the doctor involved.

A high standard of note keeping reflects a high standard of care.

When the records have been obtained from the hospital they are photocopied and the solicitor then instructs a medical expert to consider the information. A report is prepared concerning the standard of care provided. This is currently measured according to the Bolam principle. Essentially this involves a view as to whether the practice adopted would be that adopted by a responsible body of medical opinion. This allows for the fact of the art as well as the science of medicine. There may be several ways of approaching the problem, but what has to be shown for a defence is that the approach adopted would be adopted by a significant number of other reasonable people.

An additional approach, adopted in Australia and becoming more common in Britain, is to request the Guidelines or Protocols of care from the hospital concerned and ask the simple question: *Did you do what you say you do and if not what is the explanation?* It is therefore very important to have guidelines, particularly for the labour ward. These guidelines should be dated and then updated, preferably on a yearly basis. With this information the expert can recommend to the solicitor whether formulating a statement of claim should be undertaken. The statement of claim will essentially state in what respects the treatment has been considered to be inadequate and is alleged to have caused the damage.

Causation

A proven deficiency of care is not enough for a case to be successful. It also has to be shown that it was the deficiency of care and not another factor that led to the damage. In order to consider this, the advice of experts in the fields of neonatology and paediatric neurology will be sought. There are many natural factors that may result in damage to a child. The most frequent one is prematurity. In many cases this appears to have been unavoidable irrespective of the standard of care. The child may have a congenital or pre-existing abnormality. If a child has such an abnormality associated with handicap then poor management of labour or misinterpretation of the CTG may have made little difference to the outcome. A case that is strong on liability may frequently fail on causation.

Probably only about one in a hundred legal cases that are commenced go to court. A proportion will be discontinued after expert opinion has recommended that there is no case to pursue. A proportion will be settled by the defending hospital trust with a recognition that the case will be difficult to defend in court. There is a growing realism by hospital trusts that a move towards resolution sooner rather than later benefits everyone. This has also been recognized by the report to the Lord Chancellor by Lord Woolf

(Lord Justice, Master of the Rolls) entitled *Access to Justice*, 1996. Families should not suffer the stress of waiting for up to 10 years while the case goes through the system.

Every hospital should have a structured approach to risk management. There must be guidelines. Cases should be identified soon after they happen when there is a risk of complaint and litigation. An internal review should take place ensuring the notes are correct and statements taken if necessary. It is important that this should be seen as not implying disciplinary action. This is called Critical Incident Review. It is a learning process, the objective of which is to avoid avoidable factors in the future.

Litigation can be reduced by good standards of care and good communication. Surely this is something to which we should aspire even without a legal threat. A comprehensive approach to medico-legal aspects in our speciality can be found in *Safe Practice in Obstetrics and Gynaecology. A Medico-Legal Handbook.*[134]

Litigation may be avoided by good practice and good communication.

Chapter 16

Conclusion

There is little doubt that electronic fetal heart rate monitoring is likely to stay because of the uncertainties of the other methods due to technical difficulties and the limited correlation of the results obtained to the clinical outcome. Contraction monitoring is likely to be by external tocography in the majority of cases. Until a perfect method is developed to identify intrapartum hypoxia, we should learn to correlate the FHR pattern with the clinical picture in order to plan the management for each individual case. More time should be devoted to educate ourselves, residents and the midwives in FHR trace interpretation because our daily practice requires this. Failure to do so may lead to unnecessary caesarean section or result in babies with birth asphyxia due to misinterpretation of the FHR trace. The benefits of intrapartum fetal monitoring in the future depend on formal education in trace interpretation, which is sadly lacking. This should be in parallel to research in pursuit of better methods of fetal surveillance.

Cardiotocography is useful if:

1 Adequate knowledge is available to interpret the trace.
2 Its limitations are known.
3 It is used appropriately.
4 The clinical picture is incorporated.
5 Additional tests are used when in doubt.
6 *Common sense prevails.*

References

1. Macdonald D., Grant A., Sheridan-Pereira M. *et al.* (1985). The Dublin randomised controlled trial of intrapartum fetal heart rate monitoring. *Am. J. Obstet. Gynecol.*, **152**, 524–539.
2. Leveno K. J., Cunningham F. G., Nelson S. *et al.* (1986). A prospective comparison of selective and universal electronic fetal monitoring in 34,995 pregnancies. *New Eng. J. Med.*, **315**, 615–619.
3. Belizan J. M., Vittar J., Nardin J. C. *et al.* (1978). Diagnosis of intrauterine growth retardation by a simple clinical method: measurement of uterine height. *Am. J. Obstet. Gynecol.*, **131**, 643–646.
4. Bennet M. J. (1977). Antenatal fetal monitoring. In *Contemporary Obstetrics & Gynaecology* (G. V. P. Chamberlain, ed.) London: Northwood Publications Ltd, pp. 117–124.
5. Boddy K., Parboosingh I. J. T., Shepherd W. C. (1976). *A Schematic Approach to Antenatal Care.* Edinburgh: Edinburgh University.
6. Calvert P. J., Crean E. E., Newcombe R. G., Pearson J. F. (1982). Antenatal screening by measurement of symphysic fundus height. *Brit. Med. J.*, **295**, 846–849.
7. FIGO (1987). Guidelines for the use of fetal monitoring. *Int. J. Gynecol. Obstet.*, **25**, 159–167.
8. Wheeler T., Murrils A. (1978). Patterns of fetal heart rate during normal pregnancy. *Brit. J. Obstet. Gynaecol.*, **85**, 18–27.
9. Parer J. T. (1982). In defense of FHR monitoring's specificity. *Cont. Obstet. Gynaecol.*, **19**, 228–234.
10. Fleischer A., Schulman H., Jagani N. *et al.* (1982). The development of fetal acidosis in the presence of an abnormal fetal heart rate tracing. 1. The average for gestation age fetus. *Am. J. Obstet. Gynecol.*, **144**, 55–60.
11. Spencer J. A. D., Johnson P. (1986). Fetal heart rate variability changes and fetal behavioural cycles during labour. *Brit. J. Obstet. Gynaecol.*, **93**, 314–321.
12. Grant A., Elbourne D., Valentin L., Alexander S. (1989). Routine fetal movement counting and risk of antepartum late death in normally formed singletons. *Lancet*, **i**, 345–349.
13. Sadovsky E., Yaffe H., Polishuk W. Z. (1974). Fetal movements in pregnancy and urinary oestriol in prediction of impending fetal death in utero. *Israel J. Med. Sci.*, **10**, 1096–1099.
14. Sadovsky E., Yaffe H. (1973). Daily fetal movement recordings and fetal prognosis. *Obstet. Gynecol.*, **41**, 845–850.

15. Sadovsky E. (1985). Monitoring fetal movements: a useful screening test. *Cont. Obstet. Gynaecol.*, **25**, 123–127.
16. Sadovsky E., Rabinowitz R., Yaffe H. (1981). Decreased foetal movements and foetal malformations. *J. Foet. Med.*, **1**, 62–64.
17. Fong Y. S., Kuldip S., Malcus P. *et al.* (1996). Assessment of fetal health should be based on maternal perception of clusters rather than episodes of fetal movements. *J. Obstet. Gynaecol. Res.*, **22**, 299–304.
18. Stanco L. M., Rabello Y., Medearis A. L., Paul R. H. (1993). Does Doppler-detected fetal movement decrease the incidence of non-reactive nonstress tests? *Obstet. Gynaecol.*, **82**, 999–1003.
19. Patrick J., Carmichael L., Laurie C., Staples C. (1984). Accelerations of the human fetal heart rate at 38 to 40 weeks' gestational age. *Am. J. Obstet. Gynecol.*, **148**, 35–41.
20. Kubli F., Boos R., Ruttgers H. *et al.* (1977). Antepartum fetal heart rate monitoring and ultrasound in obstetrics. In *RCOG Scientific Meeting* (R. W. Beard, ed.) London: RCOG, pp. 28–47.
21. Schifrin B. S., Foye G., Amato J. *et al.* (1979). Routine fetal heart rate monitoring in the antepartum period. *Obstet. Gynecol.*, **54**, 21–25.
22. Keagan K. A., Paul R. H. (1980). Antepartum fetal heart rate monitoring: non-stress test as a primary approach. *Am. J. Obstet. Gynecol.*, **136**, 75–80.
23. Flynn A. M., Kelly J., Mansfield H. *et al.* (1982). A randomised controlled trial of non-stress antepartum cardiotocography. *Brit. J. Obstet. Gynaecol.*, **89**, 427–433.
24. Smith C. B., Phelan J. P., Paul R. H., Broussard P. (1985). Fetal acoustic stimulation testing: a retrospective experience with the fetal acoustic stimulation test. *Am. J. Obstet. Gynecol.*, **153**, 567–568.
25. Smith C. V., Phelan J. P., Platt L. D. *et al.* (1986). Acoustic stimulation testing II. A randomized clinial comparison with the non-stress test. *Am. J. Obstet. Gynecol.*, **155**, 131–134.
26. Schiff E., Lipitz S., Sivan E. *et al.* (1992). Acoustic stimulation as a diagnostic test: comparison with oxytocin challenge test. *J. Perinat. Med.*, **20**, 275–279.
27. Chamberlain P. F., Manning F. A., Morrison I. *et al.* (1984). Ultrasound evaluation of amniotic fluid (vol. 1). The relationship of marginal and decreased amniotic fluid volumes to perinatal outcome. *Am. J. Obstet. Gynecol.*, **150**, 245–249.
28. Crowley P., O'Herlihy C., Boylon P. (1984). The value of ultrasound measurement of amniotic fluid volume on the management of prolonged pregnancies. *Brit. J. Obstet. Gynaecol.*, **91**, 444–445.
29. Phelan J. P., Ahn M. O., Smith C. V. *et al.* (1987). Amniotic fluid index measurements during pregnancy. *J. Reprod. Med.*, **32**, 601–604.
30. Jeng C. J., Jou T. J., Wang K. G. *et al.* (1990). Amniotic fluid index measurements with the four quadrant technique during pregnancy. *J. Reprod. Med.*, **35**, 674–677.
31. Rutherford S. E., Phelan J. P., Smith C. V., Jacobs N. (1987). The four quadrant assessment of amniotic fluid volume: an adjunct to ante-partum fetal heart rate testing. *Obstet. Gynecol.*, **70**, 353–356.
32. Moore T. R., Cayle J. E. (1990). The amniotic fluid index in normal human pregnancy. *Am. J. Obstet. Gynecol.*, **162**, 1168–1173.

33. Moore T. R. (1990). Superiority of the four quadrant sum over the single deepest pocket technique in ultrasonographic identification of abnormal amniotic fluid volumes. *Am. J. Obstet. Gynecol.*, **163**, 762–767.

34. Rutherford S. E., Smith C. V., Phelan J. P. *et al.* (1987). Four quadrant assessment of amniotic fluid volume. Inter-observer and intra-observer variation. *J. Reprod. Med.*, **32**, 587–589.

35. Clark S. L., Sabey P., Jolly K. (1989). Nonstress testing with acoustic stimulation and amniotic fluid volume assessment: 5973 tests without unexpected fetal death. *Am. J. Obstet. Gynecol.*, **160**, 694–697.

36. Anandakumar C., Biswas A., Arulkumaran S. *et al.* (1993). Should assessment of amniotic fluid volume form an integral part of antenatal fetal surveillance of high risk pregnancy? *Aust. NZ. J. Obstet. Gynecol.*, **33**, 272–275.

37. Vintzileos A. M., Fleming A. D., Scorza W. E. *et al.* (1991). Relationship between fetal biophysical activities and cord blood gas values. *Am. J. Obstet. Gynecol.*, **165**, 707–712.

38. Manning F. A., Platt L. D., Sipos L. (1980). Antepartum fetal evaluation: development of a biophysical profile. *Am. J. Obstet. Gynecol.*, **136**, 787–790.

39. Manning F. A., Morrison I., Harman C. R. *et al.* (1987). Fetal assessment based on fetal biophysical profile scoring: experience in 19,221 referred high risk pregnancies. *Am. J. Obstet. Gynecol.*, **157**, 880–884.

40. Johnson J. M., Hareman C. R., Lange I. R., Manning F. A. (1986). Biophysical scoring in the management of postterm pregnancy: an analysis of 307 patients. *Am. J. Obstet. Gynecol.*, **154**, 269–273.

41. Eden R. D., Seifert L. S., Koack L. D. *et al.* (1988). A modified biophysical profile for antenatal fetal surveillance. *Obstet. Gynecol.*, **71**, 365–369.

42. Maeda K. (1990). Computerized analysis of cardiotocograms and fetal movements. *Baillieres Clin. Obstet. Gynaecol.*, **4**, 797–813.

43. Timor-Trisch I. E., Dierker L. J., Zador R. H., Mortimer G. R. (1978). Fetal movements associated with fetal heart rate accelerations. *Am. J. Obstet. Gynecol.*, **131**, 276–281.

44. Montan S., Arulkumaran S., Ratnam S. S. (1994). Evaluation of a simple method to assess fetal well-being in antenatal clinic. *J. Perinat. Med.*, **22**, 175–180.

45. Drew J. H., Kelly E., Chew F. T. K. *et al.* (1992). Prospective study of the quality of survival of infants with critical reserve detected by antenatal cardiotocography. *Aust. NZ. J. Obstet. Gynaecol.*, **32**, 32–35.

46. Navot D., Mor-Yosef S., Granat M., Sadovsky E. (1983). Antepartum fetal heart rate pattern associated with major congenital malformations. *Obstet. Gynecol.*, **63**, 414–417.

47. Buchdahl R., Hird M., Gibb D. *et al.* (1990). Listeriosis revisited: the role of the obstetrician. *Brit. J. Obstet. Gynaecol.*, **97**, 186–189.

48. Hobel C. J., Hyvarinen M. A., Okada D. M., Oh W. (1973). Prenatal and intrapartum high risk screening. 1. Prediction of the high risk neonate. *Am. J. Obstet. Gynecol.*, **117**, 1–9.

49. Arulkumaran S., Gibb D. M. F., Ratnam S. S. (1983). Experience with a selective intrapartum fetal monitoring policy. *Sing. J. Obstet. Gynecol.*,

14, 47–51.

50. Ingemarsson I., Arulkumaran S., Ingemarsson E. *et al.* (1986). Admission test: a screening test for fetal distress in labour. *Obstet. Gynecol.*, **68**, 800–806.

51. Malcus P., Gudmundson S., Marsal K. *et al.* (1991). Umbilical artery Doppler velocimetry as a labour admission test. *Obstet. Gynecol.*, **77**, 10–16.

52. Sarno A. P. J., Ahn M. O., Brar H. *et al.* (1989). Intrapartum Doppler velocimetry, amniotic fluid volume and fetal heart rate as predictors of subsequent fetal distress. *Am. J. Obstet. Gynecol.*, **161**, 1508–1511.

53. Chauchan S. P., Washburne J. F., Magann E. F. *et al.* (1995). A randomized study to assess the efficacy of the amniotic fluid index as a fetal admission test. *Obstet. Gynecol.*, **86**, 9–13.

54. Teoh T. G., Gleeson R. P., Darling M. R. (1992). Measurement of amniotic fluid volume in early labour is a useful admission test. *Brit. J. Obstet. Gynaecol.*, **99**, 859–860.

55. Chua S., Arulkumaran S., Kurup A. *et al.* (1996). Search for the most predictive tests of fetal well-being in early labour. *J. Perinat. Med.*, **24**, 199–206.

56. Chan F. Y., Lam C., Lam Y. H. *et al.* (1994). Umbilical artery Doppler velocimetry compared with fetal heart rate monitoring as a labor admission test. *Eur. J. Obstet. Gynecol. Reprod. Biol.*, **54**, 1–6.

57. Keegan K. A. J., Waffarn F., Quilligan E. J. (1985). Obstetric characteristics and fetal heart rate patterns of infants who convulse during the newborn period. *Am. J. Obstet. Gynecol.*, **153**, 732–737.

58. Van der Merwe P., Gerretsen G., Visser G. (1985). Fixed heart rate pattern after intrauterine accidental decerebration. *Obstet. Gynecol.*, **65**, 125–127.

59. Menticoglou S. M., Manning F. A., Harman C. R., Morrison I. (1989). Severe fetal brain injury without evident intrapartum trauma. *Obstet. Gynecol.*, **74**, 457–461.

60. Schields J. R., Schifrin B. S. (1988). Perinatal antecedents of cerebral palsy. *Obstet. Gynecol.*, **71**, 899–905.

61. Leveno K. J., William M. L., De Palma R. T., Whalley P. J. (1983). Perinatal outcome in the absence of antepartum fetal heart rate accelerations. *Obstet. Gynecol.*, **61**, 347–355.

62. Devoe L. D., McKenzie J., Searle N. S., Sherline D. M. (1985). Clinical sequelae of the extended non-stress test. *Am. J. Obstet. Gynecol.*, **151**, 1074–1078.

63. Brown R., Patrick J. (1981). The non-stress test: how long is long enough? *Am. J. Obstet. Gynecol.*, **141**, 646–651.

64. Phelan J. P., Ahn M. O. (1994). Perinatal observations in forty-eight neurologically impaired term infants. *Am. J. Obstet. Gynecol.*, **171**, 424–431.

65. Herbst A., Ingemarsson I. (1994). Intermittent versus continuous electronic fetal monitoring in labour. *Brit. J. Obstet. Gynaecol.*, **101**, 663–668.

66. Arulkumaran S., Yeoh S. C., Gibb D. M. F. *et al.* (1985). Obstetric outcome of meconium stained liquor in labour. *Sing. Med. J.*, **26**, 523–526.

67. Steer P. J. (1985). Fetal distress. In *Risks of Labour* (J. Crawford, ed.) Chichester: John Wiley & Sons, pp. 11–31.
68. Montan S., Solum T., Sjoberg N. O. (1984). Influence of the β-1 adrenoceptor blocker atenolol on antenatal cardiotocography. *Acta Obstet. Gynecol. Scand.*, **118**, 99–102.
69. Melchior J., Bernard N. (1989). Second stage fetal heart rate patterns. In *Fetal Monitoring – Physiology and Techniques of Antenatal and Intrapartum Assessment* (J. A. D. Spencer, ed.) Tunbridge Wells: Castle House Publications, pp. 155–158.
70. Arulkumaran S., Yang M., Chia Y. T., Ratnam S. S. (1991). Reliability of intrauterine pressure measurements. *Obstet. Gynecol.*, **78**, 800–802.
71. Caldeyro B. R., Sica-Blanco Y., Poseiro J. J. *et al.* (1957). A quantitative study of the action of synthetic oxytocin on the pregnant human uterus. *J. Pharmacol.*, **121**, 18–31.
72. Hon E. H., Paul R. H. (1973). Quantitation of uterine activity. *Obstet. Gynecol.*, **42**, 368–370.
73. Steer P. J. (1977). The measurement and control of uterine contractions. In *The Current Status of Fetal Heart Rate Monitoring and Ultrasound in Obstetrics* (R. W. Beard, ed.). London: RCOG Press, pp. 48–68.
74. Gibb D. M. F. (1993). Measurement of uterine activity in labour – clinical aspects. *Brit. J. Obstet. Gynaecol.*, **110**, 28–31.
75. Arulkumaran S., Gibb D. M. F., Ratnam S. S. *et al.* (1985). Total uterine activity in induced labour – an index of cervical and pelvic tissue resistance. *Brit. J. Obstet. Gynaecol.*, **92**, 693–697.
76. Arulkumaran S., Chua S., Chua T. M. *et al.* (1991). Uterine activity in dysfunctional labour and target uterine activity to be aimed with oxytocin titration. *Asia Oceania J. Obstet. Gynaecol.*, **17**, 101–106.
77. Chua S., Kurup A., Arulkumaran S., Ratnam S. S. (1990). Augmentation of labor: does internal tocography produce better obstetric outcome than external tocography? *Obstet. Gynecol.*, **76**, 164–167.
78. Beckley S., Gee H., Newton J. R. (1991). Scar rupture in labour after previous lower segment caesarean section: the role of uterine activity measurement. *Brit. J. Obstet. Gynaecol.*, **98**, 265–269.
79. Arulkumaran S., Chua S., Ratnam S. S. (1992). Symptoms and signs with scar rupture: value of uterine activity measurements. *Aust. NZ. J. Obstet. Gynaecol.*, **32**, 208–212.
80. Gibb D. M. F., Arulkumaran S. (1987). Assessment of uterine activity. In *Clinics in Obstetrics and Gynaecology* (M. Whittle, ed.). London: Bailliere Tindall, pp. 111–130.
81. Arulkumaran S., Ingemarsson I. (1990). Appropriate technology in intrapartum fetal surveillance. In *Progress in Obstetrics and Gynaecology* (J. W. W. Studd, ed.). Edinburgh: Churchill Livingstone, pp. 127–140.
82. Ingemarsson I., Arulkumaran S., Ratnam S. S. (1985). Single injection of terbutaline in term labor. 1. Effect on fetal pH in cases with prolonged bradycardia. *Am. J. Obstet. Gynecol.*, **153**, 859–865.
83. Ingemarsson I., Arulkumaran S., Ratnam S. S. (1985). Single injection of terbutaline in term labor. 2. Effect on uterine activity. *Am. J. Obstet. Gynecol.*, **153**, 865–869.
84. Sica B. Y., Sala N. L. (1961). Oxytocin. In *Proceedings of an International Symposium London* (R. Caldeyro-Barcia and H. Heller, eds), Oxford:

Pergamon Press, pp. 127–136.

85. Arulkumaran S., Ratnam S. S. (1988). Caesarean sections in the management of severe hypertensive disorders in pregnancy and eclampsia. *Sing. J. Obstet. Gynaecol.*, **19**, 61–66.

86. Modanlou H. D., Freeman R. H. (1982). Sinusoidal fetal heart rate patterns; its definition and clinical significance. *Am. J. Obstet. Gynecol.*, **142**, 1033–1038.

87. Arulkumaran S., Tham K. F. (1988). Sinusoidal like fetal heart rate pattern – real time ultrasound may help in differential diagnosis. *Acta Obstet. Gynaecol. Scand.*, **67**, 573.

88. Gray J. H., Dumore D. W., Luther E. R. (1978). Sinusoidal fetal heart rate pattern associated with alphaprodine administration. *Obstet. Gynecol.*, **52**, 678–679.

89. Arulkumaran S., Wong Y. C., Anandakumar C., Ratnam S. S. (1989). Sinusoidal like pattern associated with acute fetomaternal transfusion. *Aust. NZ. J. Obstet. Gynaecol.*, **29**, 364–365.

90. Boylan P. (1985). Sinusoidal-like tracing in fetus with rhesus hemolytic anemia. *Am. J. Obstet. Gynecol.*, **145**, 892–893.

91. Beard R. W., Morris E. D., Clayton S. G. (1967). pH of fetal capillary blood as an indicator of the condition of the fetus. *J. Obstet. Gynaecol. Brit. Cwlth.*, **74**, 812–817.

92. Beard R. W., Filshie G. M., Knight C. A., Roberts G. M. (1971). The significance of the changes in the continuous fetal heart rate in the first stage of labour. *J. Obstet. Gynaecol. Br. Cwlth.*, **78**, 865–881.

93. Ingemarsson E. (1981). Routine electronic fetal monitoring during labor. *Acta Obstet. Gynaecol. Scand.*, **99**, 1–29.

94. Zalor R. W., Quilligan E. J. (1979). The influence of scalp sampling on the caesarean section rate for fetal distress. *Am. J. Obstet. Gynecol.*, **135**, 239–246.

95. Katz M., Mazor M., Insler V. (1981). Fetal heart rate patterns and scalp pH as predictors of fetal distress. *Israel J. Med. Sci.*, **17**, 260–265.

96. Paul R. H., Suidan A. K., Yeh S. Y. *et al.* (1975). Clinical fetal monitoring. VII. The evaluation and significance of intrapartum baseline variability. *Am. J. Obstet. Gynecol.*, **123**, 206–210.

97. Schifrin B. S., Dame L. (1972). Fetal heart rate patterns: prediction of Apgar score. *JAMA*, **219**, 1322–1325.

98. Starks G. C. (1980). Correlation of meconium stained amniotic fluid, early intrapartum fetal pH and Apgar scores as predictors of perinatal outcome. *Obstet. Gynecol.*, **55**, 604–609.

99. Sykes G. S., Johnson P., Ashworth F. *et al.* (1982). Do Apgar scores indicate asphyxia? *Lancet*, **i**, 494–496.

100. Nordstrom L., Arulkumaran S., Chua S. *et al.* (1995). Continuous maternal glucose infusion during labor: effects on maternal and fetal glucose and lactate lends. *Am. J. Perinatol.*, **12**, 357–362.

101. Huch A., Huch R., Rooth G. (1994). Guidelines for blood sampling and measurements of pH and blood gas values in obstetrics. *Eur. J. Obstet. Gynecol. Reprod. Biol.*, **54**, 165–175.

102. Ingemarsson I., Ingemarsson E., Solum T., Westgren M. (1980). Influence of occiput posterior position on the fetal heart rate pattern. *Obstet. Gynecol.*, **55**, 301–306.

103. Clarke S. L., Gimovsky M. L., Miller F. C. (1983). Fetal heart rate response to scalp blood sampling. *Am. J. Obstet. Gynecol.*, **144**, 706–708.
104. Clarke S. L., Gimovsky M. L., Miller F. C. (1984). The scalp stimulation test: a clinical alternative to fetal scalp blood sampling. *Am. J. Obstet. Gynecol.*, **148**, 274–277.
105. Arulkumaran S., Ingemarsson I., Ratnam S. S. (1987). Fetal heart rate response to scalp stimulation as a test for fetal wellbeing in labour. *Asia Oceania J. Obstet. Gynaecol.*, **13**, 131–135.
106. Edersheim T. G., Hutson J. M., Druzin M. L., Kogut E. A. (1987). Fetal heart rate response to vibratory acoustic stimulation predicts fetal pH in labor. *Am. J. Obstet. Gynecol.*, **157**, 1557–1560.
107. Fisk N. M., Nicolaidis P., Arulkumaran S. *et al.* (1991). Vibroacoustic stimulation is not associated with sudden fetal catecholamine release. *Early Hum. Dev.*, **25**, 11–17.
108. Arulkumaran S., Skurr B., Tong H. *et al.* (1991). No evidence of hearing loss due to fetal acoustic stimulation test. *Obstet. Gynecol.*, **78**, 283–285.
109. Spencer J. A. D., Deans A., Nicolaidis P., Arulkumaran S. (1991). Fetal response to vibroacoustic stimulation during low and high fetal heart rate variability episodes in late pregnancy. *Am. J. Obstet. Gynecol.*, **165**, 86–90.
110. Clarke S. L., Paul R. H. (1985). Intrapartum fetal surveillance: the role of fetal scalp blood sampling. *Am. J. Obstet. Gynecol.*, **153**, 717–720.
111. Ingemarsson I., Arulkumaran S. (1989). Reactive FHR response to sound stimulation in fetuses with low scalp blood pH. *Brit. J. Obstet. Gynaecol.*, **96**, 562–565.
112. Irion O., Stuckelberger P., Montquin J. M. *et al.* (1996). Is intrapartum vibratory acoustic stimulation a valid alternative to fetal scalp pH determination. *Brit. J. Obstet. Gynaecol.*, **103**, 642–647.
113. Recommendations arising from the 26th RCOG study group (1993). In *Intrapartum Fetal Surveillance* (J. A. D. Spencer, ed.). London: RCOG Press, pp. 387–393.
114. Dunphy B. C., Robinson J. N., Sheil O. M. *et al.* (1991). Caesarean section for fetal distress, the interval from decision to delivery, and the relative risk of poor neonatal condition. *Brit. J. Obstet. Gynecol.*, **11**, 241–244.
115. Gillmer M. D. G., Combe D. (1979). Intrapartum fetal monitoring practice in the United Kingdom. *Brit. J. Obstet. Gynaecol.*, **86**, 753–758.
116. Wheble A. M., Gillmer M. D. G., Spencer J. A. D., Sykes G. S. (1989). Changes in fetal monitoring practice in the UK: 1977–1984. *Brit. J. Obstet. Gynaecol.*, **96**, 1140–1147.
117. Rosen K. G., Dagbjartsson A., Henriksson B. A. *et al.* (1984). The relationship between circulating catecholamine and ST waveform in the fetal lamb electrocardiogram during hypoxia. *Am. J. Obstet. Gynecol.*, **149**, 190–195.
118. Lilja H., Arulkumaran S., Lindecrantz K. *et al.* (1988). Fetal ECG during labour; a presentation of a micro-processor based system. *J. Biomed. Eng.*, **10**, 348–350.

119. Arulkumaran S., Lilja H., Lindecrantz K. *et al.* (1990). Fetal ECG waveform analysis should improve fetal surveillance in labour. *J. Perinat. Med.*, **187**, 13–22.
120. MacLachlan N. A., Harding K., Spencer J. A. D., Arulkumaran S. (1991). Fetal heart rate, fetal acidaemia and the T/QRS ratio of the fetal ECG in labour. *Brit. J. Obstet. Gynaecol.*, **99**, 26–31.
121. Westgate J., Harris M., Curnow J. S. H., Greene K. R. (1992). Randomised trial of cardiotocography alone or with ST waveform analysis for intrapartum monitoring. *Lancet*, **ii**, 194–198.
122. Raymond S. P. W, Whitfield C. R. (1979). Systolic time intervals of the fetal cardiac cycle. *Clin. Obstet. Gynecol.*, **1**, 85–201.
123. Hon E. H., Koh K. S. (1979). Electromechanical intervals of the fetal cardiac cycle. *Clin. Obstet. Gynecol.*, **6**, 215–221.
124. Organ L. W., Bernstein A., Smith K. C., Rowe I. H. (1974). The pre-ejection period of the fetal heart: patterns of change during labour. *Am. J. Obstet. Gynecol.*, **120**, 49–55.
125. Hon E. H., Murata Y., Zanini B. *et al.* (1974). Continuous microfilm display of the electromechanical intervals of the cardiac cycle. *Obstet. Gynecol.*, **43**, 722–728.
126. Johnson N., Johnson V. A., Fisher J. *et al.* (1991). Fetal monitoring with pulse oximetry. *Brit. J. Obstet. Gynaecol.*, **98**, 36–41.
127. Trudinger B. J., Giles W. B., Cook C. M. (1985). Flow velocity waveforms in the maternal uteroplacental and umbilical placental circulation. *Am. J. Obstet. Gynecol.*, **152**, 155–163.
128. Laurin J., Marsal K., Persson P. H., Lingman G. (1987). Ultrasound measurements of fetal blood flow in predicting fetal outcome. *Brit. J. Obstet. Gynaecol.*, **94**, 940–948.
129. Malcus P., Hokegard K. H., Kjellmer I. *et al.* (1991). The relationship between atrial blood velocity waveforms and acid base status in the fetal lamb during experimental asphyxia. *Int. J. Maternal Fetal Invest.*, **1**, 29–34.
130. Ingemarsson I., Arulkumaran S. (1986). Fetal acid base balance in low risk patients in labour. *Am. J. Obstet. Gynecol.*, **155**, 66–69.
131. Dawes G. S., Redman C. W. G., Smith J. H. (1985). Improvements in the registration and analysis of fetal heart records at the bedside. *Brit. J. Obstet. Gynaecol.*, **92**, 317–325.
132. Cheng L. C., Gibb D. M. F., Ayaji R., Soothill P.W. (1992). A comparison between computerised (mean range) and clinical visual cardiotocographic assessment. *Brit. J. Obstet. Gynaecol.*, **99**, 817–820.
133. Keith R. D. F., Beckley S., Garibaldi J. M., Westgate J. A. *et al.* (1995). A multicentre comparative study of 17 experts and an intelligent computer system for managing labour using the cardiotocogram. *Brit. J. Obstet. Gynaecol.*, **102**, 688–700.
134. Clements R. V. (1995). *Safe Practice in Obstetrics and Gynaecology. A Medico-Legal Handbook.* Edinburgh: Churchill Livingstone.

Index

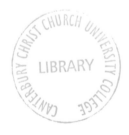